THE SIMPLE SCIENCE OF WELLNESS

THE
SIMPLE
SCIENCE
OF WELLNESS

HARNESS THE POWER WITHIN FOR A FULL INNATE TRANSFORMATION

FIT
5·40·5

GAVIN SINCLAIR &
RYAN COPLESTON

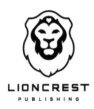

LIONCREST
PUBLISHING

THE SIMPLE SCIENCE OF WELLNESS
Harness the Power Within for a Full Innate Transformation

ISBN 978-1-5445-2127-5 *Hardcover*
      978-1-5445-1354-6 *Paperback*
      978-1-5445-1353-9 *Ebook*

We dedicate this book to all those on the journey to better health.

CONTENTS

INTRODUCTION

Derek is on the run. He works a full-time job as a bus driver and often picks up additional shifts to earn extra money for his family. He's been sitting behind the wheel for thirteen years, doing a job that's so sedentary he rarely gets any exercise, and keeps him so busy he almost never has time to stop and eat a proper meal. He eats whatever is quick and convenient, often at the expense of quality. At forty-two years old, his blood sugar rides this roller-coaster with him, and he's significantly overweight. He also smokes and doesn't sleep well.

It hasn't always been this way—when Derek was younger, he played soccer and was quite healthy and fit. Once he began working, however, he didn't have much time for physical activity. After his daughter was born, time was so tight that hitting the gym didn't even seem like an option.

Now he's struggling with pain in his knees and lower back and has headaches almost daily. He's prediabetic and also has psoriasis and high blood pressure. It seems like the only thing he *doesn't* have is an official diagnosis for any of these problems. Nonetheless, he's definitely a ticking time bomb.

Derek has tried to change things. He lost a bit of weight with a popular weight-loss program, and if he had continued, he most likely would have lost more. The calorie-counting program, however, didn't promote a change in lifestyle, which was what he desperately needed. The fitness programs he tried were similarly unsustainable: they all required too drastic a change or pushed toward seemingly unattainable, unsustainable goals. A personal trainer seemed like a good solution, but Derek wasn't able to fit the workout sessions into his busy schedule. He didn't think he would have made much progress anyway, due to his back pain.

Just recently, Derek noticed that he had trouble breathing when walking up flights of stairs, and this was a wake-up call for him. He realized that if he didn't do something to change, he might not be around to see his daughter grow up.

Derek is not alone. You may recognize some parts of his story in your own life; after all, more and more of us struggle with chronic illness and other challenges to our physical and mental well-being than ever before.

If Derek's story doesn't strike a chord, you may recognize yourself in Lynn, a team leader who works in a demanding corporate setting, has two kids, and plenty of stress. Like many mothers, she puts the needs of others above her own and is always striving to achieve that elusive work/life balance. The balance is tough to maintain, which only amplifies Lynn's stress. This elevated level of stress makes her feel "tired but wired" at the end of her day—she struggles to switch off and rarely sleeps well.

Lynn knows her lifestyle is taking a toll. Physically, she suffers from chronic headaches, and she has developed irritable bowel issues. Emotionally, she has noticed that her fuse is getting shorter. She's dismayed that she gets upset with her so kids easily, and often gives unwarranted, angry responses. She feels on edge most of the time, and it seems increasingly likely that she might have an emotional meltdown. On a good day, she has just enough energy to accomplish her tasks for the day, but when night rolls around, she's got nothing left. While she recognizes the immediate mental and emotional effects of her stressful lifestyle, she may not realize she's creating chronic inflammation in her body—a precursor to long-term health problems.

Lynn is young, but she can't assume that this stress won't

be the catalyst for heart disease. This is now the leading cause of death in women in the United States, of which two-thirds suffer sudden death with no prior symptoms.[1] [2] She's also at risk for cancer, since we know that an estimated 90 to 95 percent of cancers are caused by the environment and a poor lifestyle. Cancer is also a leading cause of death for people under the age of sixty—Lynn is not immune.[3]

Nobody is.

THE REALITY OF CHRONIC ILLNESS

Unfortunately, lifestyles like Derek's and Lynn's are becoming the norm. We pound the pavement all day, and then, without stopping to take a breath, we tackle the seemingly endless list of responsibilities that greet us when we get home. This is especially true when we have young children who need constant care; our personal time seems to evaporate during these years. Usually during this season of life, we think it's impossible to prioritize our health and wellness. No matter our age, though, many of us struggle

1   Jiaquan Xu et al., "Deaths: Final Data for 2013," *National Vital Statistics Report* 64, no. 2 (Feb. 16, 2016): 1–119.

2   Véronique L. Roger et al., "Heart Disease and Stroke Statistics—2012 Update," *Circulation* 125, no. 1 (December 15, 2011). https://doi.org/10.1161/CIR.0b013e31823ac046.

3   Preetha Anand et al., "Cancer Is a Preventable Disease That Requires Major Lifestyle Changes," *Pharmaceutical Research* 25 (July 2008): 2097–2116. https://link.springer.com/ article/10.1007%2Fs11095-008-9661-9.

with health and wellness challenges. Even worse, most of us don't feel empowered to address them ourselves.

When we experience stress on a regular basis, we may not even recognize what's going on. Many of us deny or are simply unaware that we're in a state of chronic stress, when in fact, we are. We figure that if we aren't literally pulling our hair out, we must be fine. That's simply not true. Even low-grade stress will lead to sickness and disease if experienced over a long period of time; the symptoms just don't manifest right away. The body is quite resilient, but we can't take that for granted because ultimately, we will always lose to a toxic lifestyle. Don't wait for symptoms to appear—if you do, there will be an uphill climb to restore your health.

The sad truth is, our lifestyles are the predominant cause of chronic illnesses, and we can be ill without knowing it. For example, insulin resistance can be present for many years before we're even aware of it, because the initial symptoms are subtle: fatigue, irritability, and weight gain don't necessarily raise red flags. However, if you remain in this suboptimal state of health, you create more disease in the body—I don't necessarily mean disease in the conventional sense, but rather a "lack of ease," or a lack of homeostasis.

The evidence is clear: diseases related to lifestyle are on

the rise. For example, a study conducted in 2015 reported that 58 percent of women and 68 percent of men over the age of forty-five in the United Kingdom (UK) were overweight or obese. Also, 3.7 million UK adults had type 2 diabetes, one in ten children were obese by the age of five, and one in five children were overweight or obese by the age of eleven.[4] Those alarming numbers are only the beginning; they are expected to increase significantly in the years to come.

NO QUICK FIXES

I believe most people want to be healthy, but when we're stressed and feel like we're short on time, the last thing we want to do is add a major new effort to our days. By nature, we look for the shortest, easiest path to our goals. We want a quick fix—an external solution to an internal problem so we can "deal with it" and just keep doing what we've always done. Unfortunately, the easiest route is usually the most dangerous or costly one in the long run.

Quick solutions appear to be easy only because we've been *conditioned* to believe in them. For instance, we see commercials for medications every day, so we believe a pill will conveniently fix our problems with very little effort

---

4   Carl Baker, "Obesity Statistics," House of Commons Library, Briefing Paper 3336 (March 20, 2018). https://www.activematters.org/wp-content/uploads/pdfs/Obesity_Statistics_ March_2018.pdf.

required. However, the most readily available information, like what we see in advertising, is not necessarily the information we *need*—at best it's insufficient, and at worst it's false. As a result, we don't truly understand what is required to establish and maintain health.

Some people come into my practice thinking they're making good choices for their health, when in fact, they are not. If they work a sedentary job, they may try to counter that inactivity with one or two workouts a week, which is admirable, but insufficient. Most are experiencing some form of stress—be it chemical, physical, emotional, or any combination of the three—but they insist or assume they're fine; there seems to be a general acceptance that these issues are just a part of life. The ongoing stress seems "normal" because so many people experience it, but that doesn't make it acceptable, at least not as far as your health is concerned. Issues resulting in ongoing stress need to be resolved, or minimized at the very least, before your health is compromised.

Other people I see are always moving at a hectic pace without considering the long-term consequences of this lifestyle. Still, others do their best to eat healthy, but they don't really know what foods to eat, or how much, or how often. They all have the best intentions but make ill-informed or poor decisions due to misinformation.

BETTER INFORMATION

From a young age, I received a different message about promoting and maintaining health than most. As a child of a chiropractor, I grew up understanding that the body is able to take care of itself. I never took an antibiotic as a young child; in fact, my siblings and I never received any medicine unless it was absolutely necessary. Our dad gave us regular chiropractic adjustments as part of our healthy living routine, helping to make us more resilient to our environments. My family didn't follow a conventional approach to health, but we also didn't have a strict or extreme lifestyle by any means—we definitely treated ourselves when we felt like it. Still, we rested when we were sick, and our parents helped us keep up on our nutrition. From a young age, we understood that we should employ these methods to help us get well when we were sick, and we should also use them to *stay* well.

My lessons in healthcare extended beyond my home life, as well. I visited my dad's office often and observed every aspect of what it meant to be a chiropractor. I watched him adjust patients, but I also paid attention to his interactions with them: he was kind and compassionate, and in turn, they respected him. Innately, I always knew I wanted to be a chiropractor—it felt natural for me to follow in my dad's footsteps. I attended chiropractic college, and later my brother and sister did the same. After college, my siblings took over my dad's practice in Canada while

I stayed in the UK, specifically Scotland, where I started my chiropractic career.

HEAL THYSELF

Running a clinic wasn't always easy. I often felt like I was being pulled from pillar to post, and it only got more intense after my first child came along. Time was at a premium, and unfortunately, diet and exercise went out the window. I stopped looking after myself, and it wasn't long before I experienced some of the same symptoms my patients had. I couldn't settle down for sleep at night, and when I did sleep, I slept poorly. Like Lynn, I was "tired but wired." I also gained weight, and that was extremely bothersome because I was typically fit. I felt lethargic, and for the first time ever, albeit mild, I developed irritable bowel issues.

My practice continued to grow, and as I spent more time helping others with their health, my own health took a backseat. I took over another clinic, and I often worked there until nine or ten o'clock at night. Patients continued to show up at that late hour, and I didn't want to turn anyone away. I relocated the clinic to a larger space to meet the growing demand, and as a result, I continued to work long hours. Again, the focus on my own health would be lacking.

Then, in my mid-thirties, I decided I couldn't continue at

my current pace—I made changes, hired more people, and lightened my load at the clinic. I was able to give myself more time to prioritize my health. I knew I wanted to live a healthier lifestyle, but I didn't have a lot of time for exercise; I had to design a program for myself that was efficient, effective, and adaptable.

That's when I focused my attention on high-intensity interval training (HIIT) and began learning how it influenced the hormones of the body. I also expanded my knowledge of nutrition and started to follow a Paleo diet. I took many factors into consideration, kept an open mind, and designed a personal program based on my findings. It worked!

Then, I had an idea. If this program worked so well for me, it might just work for my patients. After all, they had similar problems. Inspired, I decided to make an offer on an empty space next to the new clinic and began offering the program as an addition to my practice. We could now offer a more well-rounded approach to care, addressing key lifestyle factors to influence and promote health.

REFINING THE PROGRAM

I was excited about my new endeavor, so I consulted my siblings, a personal development coach, and one of my associate chiropractors, Ryan (who is the co-author of this book), to further develop and refine the program. As a group, we had more than fifty years of combined clinical experience to draw from, and we focused on identifying the most common health concerns of our clients and patients. It was no surprise that high blood pressure, arthritis, and obesity topped the list. We also identified the challenges that frequently held people back from achieving their ideal life and health—time, energy, and fluctuating moods were common themes.

To address these concerns, we drew from our experience and the most up-to-date scientific research to create a program called FIT 5-40-5. FIT is an acronym for *Full Innate Transformation*, and 5-40-5 summarizes the program specifics, which we'll get into shortly.

FIT 5-40-5 is clear, concise, and simple; you can easily implement it to transform your health. It leads to weight loss, increased muscle tone, improved mood, more energy and vitality, decreased stress, and better nutrition. It also provides you with effective tools, processes, and guidance to ensure that your optimal health goals become reality. The program can help you look and feel better than you have in years, or maybe even better than ever!

BALANCE FOR OPTIMAL HEALTH

FIT 5-40-5 combines three vital components of

health—exercise, nutrition, and mindfulness—into one easy-to-follow program. Think of these components as the legs of a three-legged stool: if one is missing, the stool cannot stand. These three components hold equal significance, and all of them must be in balance for optimal health.

For some, this is self-evident. However, for others, their attempts at improving health might only focus on diet, exercise, or meditation as stand-alone methods—neglecting or failing to realize that the other two components are necessary parts of the whole picture. Movement affects our state of mind, just as diet affects the function of the brain and our ability to move—we can't give one aspect more attention than the others, and we can't rely on the hope that one will be strong enough to compensate for weakness or lack in the other two. If the only thing I do to take care of myself is exercise, I might get some results, and I might even look great, but it won't lead to optimal health. If there's emotional stress in the house and I'm eating a terrible diet, my body will eventually succumb to chronic stress, no matter how much I exercise.

FIT 5-40-5 focuses on these three main components to help you get control of your life and health! We will dig deep into each component in later chapters, but for now, here's a preview:

The first key component of FIT 5-40-5 is exercise. As I mentioned earlier, it's based on the principles of HIIT, which uses exercises that incorporate total body movement. We adapt the exercises based on the needs of the individual, changing certain variables so every participant can move toward optimal health and fitness results. We create workouts so that each person gets the benefits of HIIT, with subtle additions to account for its shortcomings (more about this later).

The core workouts of FIT 5-40-5 consist of 40-second bursts of 5 exercises, repeated 5 times, with a one-minute break between intervals. The bursts are a bit longer than conventional HIIT, but we still maintain a short timeframe for training.

We use HIIT for fitness because it's extremely efficient, and it's effective in breaking down and burning fat. This full-body workout releases catecholamines (adrenaline, norepinephrine, and dopamine), increases blood flow to all areas of the body, particularly those that get the most use, and achieves a fat-burning advantage. In addition, the adrenaline increase it produces can facilitate some appetite suppression.[5] [6] There are many other benefits

---

5   Michael Wewege et al., "The Effects of High-Intensity Interval Training vs. Moderate-Intensity Continuous Training on Body Composition in Overweight and Obese Adults: A Systematic Review and Meta-Analysis," *Obesity Reviews* 18, no. 6 (April 11, 2017): 635-646. https://doi.org/10.1111/obr.12532.

6   Andrea Nicolò and Michele Girardi, "The Physicology of Interval Training: A New Target to HIIT," *The Journal of Physiology* 594, no. 24 (Dec. 15, 2016): 7169-7170. https://dx.doi.org/10.1113%2FJP273466.

of HIIT, all of which address the most common health problems we face today. We'll discuss all of this in more detail in Chapter 3: Movement, Fitness, and Exercise.

THE SECOND COMPONENT: NUTRITION

The second key component of FIT 5-40-5 is nutrition. In the flagship transformation program, we practice the eating habit of *grazing*, or consuming smaller portions of food throughout the day. Eating food in this manner has many benefits for our physiology and body functions—it helps us maintain a higher metabolism, helps the body use energy more efficiently, overcomes weight-loss resistance, and makes us more effective at burning fat.

Of course, more importantly than knowing when to eat, is knowing *what* to eat. This is where Ryan's passion lies, and he will tell you a bit more about his story in section three. Our nutrition component is formulated by our "Core 40 Food Guide." This is made up of five different food groups with eight foods per group, which ensures you consume a great variety of real, whole, nutrient-dense foods.

As we discussed earlier, inflammation can lead to chronic illnesses such as heart disease, diabetes, and cancer—for that reason, we focus on the consumption of inflammation-reducing foods. The familiar phrase "Let thy food be thy medicine" definitely describes our philosophy of nutrition.

Our goal is to help you fuel your body so you can perform at your best, while also drastically reducing your risk of chronic disease.

You might have had trouble adhering to nutrition plans in the past because they were too rigid, or they didn't take into account your individual likes and dislikes. Our system is different, because there's room for choices and variety. If you're a vegetarian, no worries, this program is easily adaptable for you! Many more details about our eating plan will come in Chapter 4.

THE THIRD COMPONENT: MINDFULNESS

The third key component of FIT 5-40-5 is mindfulness. This aspect of health is often overlooked, or at least not given the emphasis it deserves. It's crucial to focus on the relationship between your mind and body—if they aren't aligned, it will be more difficult to achieve your goals. Our personal-development coaches have created easy-to-follow meditations and visualizations to help program participants get into the right state of mind for optimal health and wellness.

For the FIT 5-40-5 mindfulness component, we recommend that you meditate for 5 minutes, followed by a breathing reflection of 40 seconds, and finishing with 5 minutes of visualization. Generally, mornings focus on energy, and evenings focus on gratitude. Depending on your needs, wants, and current lifestyle, we will help guide you in the process. (Look for more details in Chapter 5.)

WHO IS THIS BOOK FOR?

This book is for anyone who desires to be healthy, struggles to make time for exercise, and needs some guidance. It's for people who want a clear and concise program that is easy to factor into their lifestyle. It's for anyone who simply wants to improve their health, and it's also for people who want to reach peak physical fitness and optimal health through natural means. No matter what you're trying to achieve, this program can help you find and maintain health.

FIT 5-40-5 is for everyone, but it's not a one-size-fits-all program—it's customized for every individual. It's appropriate for those who are obese or struggling with their weight, yet challenging enough for more advanced athletes. No one is too far gone, nor is anyone too healthy to participate. In fact, our oldest client at the moment is eighty-nine, and he says he feels better than he did twenty years ago! Our program is designed so you can challenge yourself, test your limits, and see progress over time.

While we aim for participants to achieve optimal health in ninety days, the long-term goal is health for life. By following our recommendations and gradually making small, manageable changes on a daily basis, you will establish a new pattern of behavior and begin living a new and improved lifestyle.

The goal of this book (and this program) is to create a new awareness and connection with the innate intelligence of your body. The best medicine for healing is already inside of you! When you begin to live in a way that harmoniously and congruently produces health from the inside out, your body will take care of the rest—it will always work toward health and wellness.

We appreciate that it's challenging to establish and maintain a healthy lifestyle. While it's not easy, we tend to make it more difficult than it needs to be. We set limitations on ourselves or make excuses, and it's not only due to a lack of desire or will—it's also due to a lack of understanding. This book will explain why we recommend the changes we do, and how they will lead to positive outcomes. We are confident you'll gain a basic understanding of the human body, become empowered to make the right health decisions, and start seeing results. When you're ready, we invite you to turn the page and begin your FIT 5-40-5 journey!

PART 1

//////////////

BODY OVER MEDICINE

CHAPTER 1

////////////

YOUR INTELLIGENT BODY

Far more Wondrous than the wonders of the world are wonders of the human body...the Mind, the Eyes, the Ears, the Nose, the Mouth, the Hands and the Heart.

—RVM

Even though I was raised to understand the importance of healthy living, I have to admit that I often take my health for granted. I don't think this is uncommon. Most of us acknowledge that health is our greatest asset, yet fail to treat it as such. All too often, we don't seriously reflect upon the way we live until we're faced with a major health challenge.

If or when we do become sick, we often search for an external solution, even though the problem is happening on the *inside*. For example, we take painkillers for headaches and back pain, antacids for heartburn, and antihypertensive medications for high blood pressure. And who can blame us? We are constantly bombarded with information about the best medicines to heal this or that condition, and advertisements about "groundbreaking treatments" for potentially fatal diseases. If we believe the media, we can't help but think that our health challenges will be helped by complex treatments or medicines.

What we should focus on, instead, is our internal strengths and our power to make decisions that support those strengths. The human body is astounding—from head to toe, it's packed with amazing and highly intelligent systems that run nonstop. If we truly understand and genuinely appreciate just how miraculous that is, we will recognize how important it is to keep the body healthy. In this chapter, I'm going to take you on a virtual tour of the body to show you its innate intelligence and explain how you can harness its power to promote lifelong health and wellness.

THE BODY REVEALED

From conception to birth, human development is governed by highly intelligent processes. Throughout the nine months of human development in the womb, cells multiply exponentially, and yet each one has unique characteristics. These cells grow together to make up the organs and functioning systems of the body that are required for life. For our bodies to be healthy and perform at their optimum potential, all of these systems must constantly communicate and work harmoniously together. This system of communication and cooperation is known as *homeostasis*.

Most of us can appreciate (or at least accept) that these processes are incredible, because we aren't involved in them at all—they occur without us giving them conscious effort. However, we seem to lose sight of the fact that the innate, bodily intelligence we develop in the womb stays with us when we enter the world, and we fail to harness and embrace what we've been given. If we understood the body better, we might treat it better. To that end, here are a few amazing facts about the human body:

THE CARDIOVASCULAR SYSTEM

Consider for a moment that your body is made of an estimated fifty to seventy trillion cells, all performing specific roles during every second of every day, and they don't require any conscious thought from you to operate. For example, the cardiovascular system is highlighted by its centerpiece, the heart, which pumps roughly two thousand gallons of blood per day. That's equivalent to the amount of fuel needed to fill the average car one hundred sixty-seven times, as much as a driver uses in two to three years! All of that blood is pumped through a network of arteries, capillaries and veins, that if unraveled, would equate to *100,000 miles* in length, or four complete trips around the world!

THE RESPIRATORY SYSTEM

The human respiratory system consists of the nose, trachea, lungs, and the diaphragm. This system processes eleven thousand liters of air per day, or the amount required to fill approximately 2,200 party balloons, from which the lungs separate five hundred and fifty liters of oxygen—the amount required by the body for daily functions.

Oxygen is used in *cellular respiration*, a process that creates energy for almost every activity and function that occurs within the body. Fortunately for us, oxygen is not in short supply—it is the most abundant element on earth, making up 23 percent of the atmosphere, and 89 percent of all the earth's water. It's unlikely a random chance that the element we need most for survival is also the one of greatest quantity on the planet.

THE DIGESTIVE SYSTEM

The physical process of digestion begins in the mouth when we take a bite of food. As we chew to break food into smaller pieces to swallow, the salivary glands secrete fluid and enzymes to keep the food and digestive tract moist and assist in food breakdown. The stomach muscles mix the food with stomach acids and regulatory hormones which continue the digestive process and help kill off any unwanted bacteria that may have entered with your food.

The food gets passed along to the small intestine for absorption, with help from pancreatic enzymes and bile from the liver. This is where *macronutrients*—commonly known as carbohydrates, fats, and proteins—are absorbed and pass into the blood and lymph (a fluid that runs in our lymphatic system, which operates much like the arterial and venous systems, circulating fluids to and from our tissues), then they're transported to the liver for processing. That apple or steak you ate is now in a form that can be used throughout the body for necessary functions. That which hasn't been absorbed will continue the journey into the large intestine, and will eventually be expelled as waste.

Not to be outdone in magnificence, the gut houses trillions of bacteria, and at any given time, it is estimated that the gut is home to approximately one to two pounds of bacteria. Most of this is good bacteria that helps digest and absorb food, stimulate cell growth, improve immune function, and prevent allergies and disease. In fact, more recent research emphasizes the relationship between a healthy gut and a healthy mind by way of the "gut-brain axis."[7] This refers to the complex relationship between the nervous system and the gastrointestinal tract which communicates via nerves and various chemical messengers in the endocrine system. It emphasizes the importance of a healthy gut biome on optimal brain function, due to the production of many important hormones and neurotransmitters by this bacteria in the gut itself.

THE ENDOCRINE SYSTEM

The endocrine system consists of a group of glands that rest just below the brain, the mother of which is the pituitary gland. This system produces an estimated fifty different hormones that act as body-wide, informational chemical messengers. They constantly work to regulate sleep, growth and repair, reproduction, mood, and metabolism. For example, brain neurotransmitters stimulate the release of the hormone serotonin for mood stabilization— and dopamine, which allows us to feel reward.

Consider the pituitary-adrenal axis which stimulates the adrenal glands to release adrenaline in response to acute stress. This quickly creates a cascade of events, including increasing blood pressure and heart rate (pumping much-needed blood to the muscles), dilating pupils to heighten

---

7   John B. Furness et al., "The Enteric Nervous System and Gastrointestinal Innervation: Integrated Local and Central Control," *Advances in Experimental Medicine and Biology* 817 (June 9, 2014): 39-71. https://doi.org/10.1007/978-1-4939-0897-4_3.

awareness, expanding the lung air passages, and increasing glucose metabolism for added energy. All of this occurs as an attempt to mount a response to the stress. These are just a few of the many things the endocrine system will do to create the perfect chemical response in the body at any given time.

THE IMMUNE SYSTEM

The immune system is our guardian, protecting us against "foreign invaders." Similar to an alarm system in the home, if it detects something, like a pathogen that shouldn't be there, it sounds the alarm. The alarm system automatically notifies the response center, and the appropriate team is deployed to contain and remove the invader or pathogen. These "alarms" go off every day in the face of millions of bacteria, viruses, and microbes that we come in contact with, and the immune system largely does its job without us taking notice. It literally saves our lives.

The immune response is carried out by two very intelligent types of cells: lymphocytes and phagocytes. *Lymphocytes* create antigens to identify specific invaders and will respond by killing them off or removing them from the body. *Phagocytes* simply ingest harmful bacteria to neutralize the threat. We won't go into the deep complexity of the immune system for the purposes of this book, but please understand that this system is standing at attention all day, every day, with its sole purpose being the preservation of your life!

THE NERVOUS SYSTEM

The nervous system consists of the brain, spinal cord, and peripheral nerves, which connect the entire body. Every cell, tissue, and organ is regulated by the nervous system— it's our information superhighway, sending signals to the brain to be processed, and subsequently sending back the appropriate response. This system allows the body to respond and adapt nearly instantaneously to our external environment. The brain alone consists of over one hundred billion neurons, which is more than the number of stars in the Milky Way! These neurons can collect and transmit information throughout the body almost instantaneously.

Signals can pass along myelinated neurons in the spinal cord to our muscles at speeds of 70 to 120 meters per second. That's like running the length of a football field in one second! You can generate a thought and begin its action in less than 150 milliseconds, faster than the blink of an eye, all by way of the nervous system. The ultimate importance of this system is highlighted by the fact that both the brain and spinal cord are completely encased by bone, providing maximal protection. It's unlikely that this is a lucky design.

THE MUSCULOSKELETAL SYSTEM

The musculoskeletal system consists of 206 bones and approximately 650 muscles. The skeleton is well known for its role in supporting the body and protecting the internal organs. However, it's also crucial to survival because it's a location for blood cell production and calcium storage.

The bones in the skeleton combine to make 360 joints throughout the body. With help from the 650 muscles, these joints give us the ability to create smooth movements for all of the daily tasks we may take for granted—like walking, running, brushing our teeth, or eating and drinking. Just the relatively simple act of walking requires harmonious movement created by approximately 200 of our muscles and 60 of our bones. That's a lot of coordination to complete an activity that's done without thinking.

Also, we are born with all of the muscle fibers we will ever have. Of course, they do get bigger, and working out can make them even bigger and stronger, but what we get at birth is what we have for life. If we were able to combine the strength of all the muscles in the body of an average adult, they could pull a resistance of approximately 50,000 pounds! This cleverly designed system is relatively the same in everyone, and without it, we would be nothing more than an immovable mass of tissue on the ground.

YOU ARE YOUR BODY'S ALLY

I hope that this tour of the body helps you begin to appreciate the complex communication networks between and within its systems. They are constantly at work, striving to keep you healthy and well. If you understand the body's amazing ability to heal, grow and repair, then you will likely be more motivated to properly care for it. I believe it's time for us to respect the body and appreciate its potential—we should have more confidence in its innate abilities before reaching for painkillers and other "solutions."

Your body's main goal is to keep you alive, but sometimes it needs some help. If you continue to ask it to fight one battle after another, it will weaken over time. That means it's time to seriously consider how your actions and behaviors contribute to its function. The choices you make either encourage your body to express health or make it more difficult to do so. Do your current actions aid the body, or do they create a daily battle?

As a natural healthcare practitioner, I've noticed that providing education and encouraging awareness at the time of diagnosis can make all the difference in a patient's outcome. When a patient understands how a health goal can be achieved and why it's important, they can make measurable progress much faster than a patient who remains uninformed. Understanding adds tremendous value because it empowers the patient to take action.

Our behaviors dictate whether we are an enemy or an ally of our bodies, and in my clinical experience, it appears that we are far more often the enemy. As we move into this next chapter, we'll discuss the current state of health, our behaviors, and what we can do to create change.

CHAPTER 2

THE CURRENT STATE OF HEALTH

Health is the crown on the well person's head that only the ill person can see.

—ROBIN SHARMA

Today, we have cutting-edge science, targeted medicines, and advanced procedures to support our amazing bodies, yet chronic illness is more prevalent than ever, especially in developed countries. Chronic disease accounts for seven out of every ten deaths in the US with chronic disease rates increasing in every age category.[8] Alarmingly, prescriptions filled by Americans between 1997 and 2016

---

8   Wullianallur Raghupathi and Viju Raghupathi, "An Empirical Study of Chronic Diseases in the United States: A Visual Analytics Approach to Public Health," *International Journal of Environmental Research and Public Health* 15, no. 2 (March 2018). https://doi.org/10.3390/ijerph15030431.

rose by 85 percent from 2.4 billion to 4.5 billion.[9] Those are frightening statistics, but what's even more alarming is that things are getting worse. We've experienced vast improvements in the fight against cancer, but more and more people are dying from it. We have the ability to reduce our risk of heart disease naturally, but statins and blood pressure medications are handed out left and right. Even in the absence of high cholesterol, people take statins to *prevent* it, thus increasing their dependency on an external source.

In the past two decades, prescription drug use has doubled.[10] Adverse reactions and addictions are compromising the quality of many people's lives, and nothing highlights this issue more than the current opioid crisis. The fact is, we're doing a poor job of tackling today's health challenges.

I think it's fair to say the answer to the problem of chronic illness won't be found in a procedure, or in a quick visit to the doctor. It would be difficult to have long-term success with these approaches, because the system doesn't focus on lifestyle as an underlying cause—it simply prescribes medication to "fix" symptoms.

---

9   Robert Preidt, "Americans Taking More Prescription Drugs Than Ever," *WebMD* (August 3, 2017). https://www.webmd.com/drug-medication/news/20170803/ americans-taking-more-prescription-drugs-than-ever-survey.

10   Ibid.

Modern medicine throws money, drugs, and treatment at health problems, yet cancer, heart disease, obesity, and diabetes are all on the rise. We're clearly missing something. It's time that we shift in the way we look at our health as practitioners, and more importantly as individuals. Our health is our responsibility, and we can no longer afford to rely on others to manage it for us.

THE STRESS RESPONSE

Many people are overwhelmed at the thought of taking responsibility for their own health issues. After all, advice comes from every direction, and it can be difficult to navigate through the information. It seems almost too simple that small, modest, and consistent lifestyle changes implemented over time can have a dramatic, positive effect.

That sense of overwhelm may also come from the common, misguided belief that we are victims of our circumstances, old age, or bad genes. When we feel powerless, it makes sense to consult an expert, or someone in authority. That's why the first stop is usually the doctor's office. Of course, that's perfectly appropriate in cases of critical or advanced illness, but chronic illness prevention lies outside the walls of a medical clinic. It can only be done by establishing and maintaining a healthy body.

A healthy body must be able to rest and repair, but an

unsettling truth of the modern world is that most of us function in a heightened state of stress for prolonged periods of time. Humans were designed with a fight-or-flight response to acute stress to keep them alive during potentially life-threatening situations. It's incredible how the body immediately adapts to a threat in our environment by creating physiological changes in the body to give us the best chance for survival.

Unfortunately, no matter how big or small the stressor, the body responds to it much the same way. A process that was designed to accommodate events of short duration can persist, leaving people in more or less of a constant, low-grade, fight-or-flight state in the face of daily stressors. We may not face immediate, life-threatening stressors every day, but poor food choices, a lack of adequate movement, and emotional stress can all sustain this unhealthy response.

Given today's hectic lifestyles, it's no surprise that our nervous systems are working in overdrive—you might have major deadlines at work, you need to run one kid to football practice and another to a birthday party, you don't have enough money to pay the bills, and you're arguing with your spouse—your nervous system is trying to cope with the onslaught of many stressors. Your body doesn't care where the stress comes from; when high alert becomes the new norm, the levels of stress hormones in the body increase. When these hormones remain elevated for long periods of time, they initiate a cascade of physiological events, eventually leading to chronic disease.[11]

Stress Response	Negative Effects on the Body When Prolonged
• Increases HR	• Weight Gain/Obesity
• Increases BP	• Fatigue
• Suppresses All Non-Essential Bodily Functions: Reproduction, Digestion	• Mood Swings/Irrational Thinking
	• Cardiovascular Disease
• Suppresses Rational Thinking	• Systemic Inflammation
• Stimulates Glucose Production	• Chronic Pain
• Tightens Muscles	• Sickness and Disease
• Increases Cortisol	• Difficulty Sleeping/Relaxing
• Suppresses Growth and Repair	• Anxiety/Depression
• Suppresses Immune System	• Headaches
	• Gastrointestinal Issues: Indigestion, Reflux

HOW DID WE GET HERE?

So, how did we end up in such a state of disrepair? To begin with, most of us do the same thing, day in and day out. See if this sounds familiar:

The alarm clock blares, you get up, shower, and head to the kitchen for breakfast. On the way there, you roust the kids and get them ready for school. Everyone shuffles out the door, the kids spend the day at school, and you go to work. You come home in the evening, look after the kids,

---

11   Yun-Zi Liu, Yun-Xia Wang, and Chun-Lei Jiang, "Inflammation: The Common Pathway of Stress-Related Diseases," *Frontiers in Human Neuroscience* 11, no. 316 (June 2017). https://dx.doi.org/10.3389%2Ffnhum.2017.00316.

drive them to various functions, and eventually try to sit down with them for dinner.

You're constantly pulled in different directions by kids, stressful work environments, and household chores; by the time you've managed to meet those demands, there's not much time left to take care of yourself. If there is any time afterward, you might relax on the couch and wind down before collapsing in bed, only to wake up the next day and do it all over again. This pattern is all too common, and it's not a good one. We often find ourselves "running on empty." It's no wonder the current state of health is in shambles!

The modern lifestyle leaves little room for movement. If we asked our client base how many of them exercise on a regular basis, I'd be surprised if 20 percent could respond that they do. They often tell us, "Oh, I went for a walk today." That's fine, and sometimes it's the least we can expect from ourselves. However, is it really enough to counter the side effects of a predominantly sedentary lifestyle? More than likely, it's not!

Our hectic schedules also predispose us to making poor nutritional choices. We often eat while we're on the move, eat as quickly as we can, or sometimes not at all—we treat mealtime as if it's a brief interruption in our busy lives, often resulting in food choices that are deficient or even void of the necessary vitamins and minerals the body requires for life.

This constant stress cycle creates chronic inflammation in the body, which by design is meant to be a short-term process. When we cope with our lack of "self-time" by succumbing to exhaustion and becoming couch potatoes, we don't do anything to solve the underlying problem. It's the same when we seek an external solution by taking pills, which often seems like the only viable option in our busy lives. For some, it is even believed to be the best option. However, we can assure you, it doesn't address the root cause. Instead, it places the responsibility for our health and well-being in the hands of others, precisely at the moment when *we ourselves* need to be taking control. We need to begin making changes to move toward health and wellness, or else our situation will never improve.

THE SCAPEGOAT: OLD AGE

As I mentioned earlier, people often blame "old age" for their health issues, but in all of our university studies, we never once saw "old age" as the diagnosis for any illness. It's true that the body does age, and the longer we live, the greater chance there is for something to go wrong, but if we make the right choices, we have the ability to be healthy into our nineties and possibly beyond!

Unfortunately, dying of "old age" seems to be rare these days. Many of us have experienced someone close to us passing from cancer, a heart attack, or stroke at an age much earlier than expected. The stories of grandparents passing peacefully seem to be less and less common. More people than ever before are living to age 100 and beyond, but on the flip side, many others are dying far too young. An article in *Time* magazine stated that the average life expectancy for a human should be 115 years. Considering we currently live to about 80 years, it's fair to say we're falling way short of our potential.

GOOD HEALTH DOESN'T HAPPEN BY ACCIDENT

In short, what many people believe to be "health" is very different from true health. The common belief is that health is the absence of illness, disease, and symptoms or any other maladies, but in reality, health is about *balance*. It's homeostasis in the body on a chemical, physical, and emotional level.

On one end of the health spectrum, there is optimum health and wellness, and on the other end is sickness and disease. When we ask patients where they think they fall on the spectrum, some will choose a place in the middle, slightly closer to optimum health. If they are symptomatic, they'll lean closer to sickness. What they may not realize is that their place on the spectrum is not a random occurrence. Good health doesn't happen by chance, with age not being a main determinant. It is the result of making healthy, informed choices on a consistent basis. Just because they are on one side of the spectrum at the moment, it doesn't mean that they will be there permanently.

The reality is, every decision we make will either move our needle towards health and wellness, or in the direction of sickness and disease. Remember, change is often a slow process, so don't be fooled if you aren't seeing obvious signs of movement one way or the other. Trust us, it's happening!

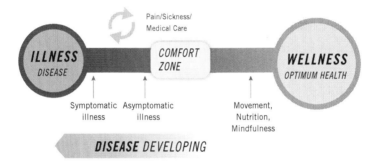

NO INSTANT CURES

In addition to believing the myth that our bodies deteriorate proportionately with old age, many of us carry beliefs that have been swayed by constant messages and marketing from big pharma and big business. These messages have a huge influence on us, and expose us to an abundance of information that isn't always true. This misinformation creates an inaccurate understanding of true health and wellness.

As previously mentioned, prescription drug use is significantly on the rise, but the overall health of the population is getting worse. It's unfortunate that today's patients expect the instant gratification of a prescription, but who can blame them? If they believe that a "quick fix" is available, then naturally, that's what they want.

The problem with the "quick fix" is that it's seldom effective, especially when the goal is prevention of chronic disease. In fact, medicine for a symptom can often contribute to the continuation of the underlying lifestyle factors that caused the problem in the first place. Can you see the problem here?

As healthcare practitioners, we are faced with this reality every day. It's not uncommon for a patient to present to us with a symptom(s) for which they have been treating with medicine(s) for months and even years, with little or no benefit. It may have been the case that there was once benefit from the medicine, but that benefit had long since ended; however, taking the medication continued. By the time many of these patients consult with us, their health challenges have often become worse over time since the causative lifestyle factors have never been addressed.

We'll say it again: the answer to a lifestyle-related health problem isn't found in a pill—it lies in transforming your lifestyle to maintain balance in the body.

HEALED BY MEDICINE

Please don't get me wrong when I urge you to steer clear of pills and medications. I think that medicine can be one of the greatest interventions we have. It saves lives every day, and it saved my life many years ago.

When I was in ninth grade, I contracted meningitis—I was seriously ill. I don't remember any of the events leading up to it, but I was in the hospital for seven days before I was coherent enough to talk with anyone. The doctor had told my parents to expect the worst—it would be a miracle if I survived, and if I did, I'd most likely have a certain degree of brain damage. He thought he might even have to amputate some fingers and toes due to a loss of circulation.

Miraculously, I pulled through with my brain and digits intact. The only medication I was given at that time was penicillin, a standard antibiotic. Two other children with meningitis were also given the medication, but sadly, they passed away. The doctor believed that since I had taken so little medication throughout my young life, the penicillin was extremely effective for me.

Our message isn't that medication is always a bad choice; that's clearly not the case. We don't want you to abuse it or take it when it's not necessary. We see this far too often in our clinics. It appears to be the easy way out, but it can negatively affect morbidity and can create a host of problems down the road.

WHICH DIRECTION WILL YOU GO?

The best prevention is not medicine, but a focus on a healthy lifestyle, and that's what the FIT 5-40-5 program is all about. Many people fail to develop this focus, either due to an overall lack of will to get healthy, a lack of understanding, or possibly both. All too often, we neglect our health until we get sick; it's only then that we realize that illness has been brewing for a long time. Had we taken preventative measures and worked to remain healthy, we wouldn't end up having to hack through a massive problem. The bottom line is that when you make better lifestyle choices, they lead you in the direction of health and wellness, rather than toward sickness and disease. It's that simple.

In Part Two of this book, we will provide information to build your confidence, and help you understand that your actions can and will create change. We will also explain our program in more detail, and help you gain a firm grasp of the fundamental science required for positive outcomes in your life.

PART 2

THE FIT 5-40-5 PROGRAM

/////////////

CHAPTER 3

MOVEMENT, FITNESS, AND EXERCISE

We do not stop exercising because we grow old, we grow old because we stop exercising!

—DR. KENNETH COOPER

We believe the conventional wisdom about fitness and exercise is bunk. Historically, it has been drilled into us that exercising three times a week is good for reducing blood pressure, lowering the risk of heart disease, and facilitating weight loss. While it's true that exercise does help to moderate these risks, it's much less beneficial if people start exercising only *after* they find out they are ill. If we exercise simply to avoid sickness, rather than to promote health and wellness, it is much less effective. As the old adage says, "prevention is easier than a cure."

Research might show that blood pressure and cholesterol decline with a certain amount of exercise, but it only tells part of the story. The falling numbers fail to shed light on the fact that the conventional goal is only to bring the numbers down to *subclinical* levels, not to optimal levels. Walking the line between subclinical and clinical means that you are in a pre-disease state, and you aren't doing enough to fully reverse it within your body—you aren't promoting health, and you definitely aren't promoting longevity.

So, what *does* help you live longer? Movement. It's precisely what your body is designed to do. However, to make a realistic and effective change, it must be specifically designed in type and duration for the purpose of optimizing the health of your body.

THE RISKS OF DIMINISHED MOVEMENT

Before we get into how increased movement can improve our health, let's take a look at what *lack* of movement costs us.

Most of us are familiar with the obvious problems associated with a lack of movement, such as weight gain, back pain, diabetes, and the risk of muscular atrophy—if you don't use your skeletal muscles, they get smaller and weaker, and eventually waste away. Decreased movement or activity also causes inflammation in the joints, which leads to *fibrosis*, the thickening of connective tissue. The poor mechanics of stiff joints result in a vicious cycle of decreased proprioception (a sense of your body in space), less stimulation to the brain, and a decrease in brain function and health.

Another consequence of inactivity is that it places undue stress on the spine—the average person who sits at a desk all day tends to have a slouched posture. We also see what has been more recently termed "text neck" in many people, due to all of the time spent hunched over and staring at screens. We realize that screen time is a part of life today, and many careers require that we spend time in front of them, but we need to take preventative measures before this stereotypical forward head posture becomes a more serious problem.

Desk workers who sit for long periods of time develop slightly rounded shoulders, a forward head carriage, and a slight curling of the back. This is not healthy or natural, but many people feel comfortable in this posture—they've been slouching for so long that the muscles required to sit up straight have atrophied from lack of use. And not only that, bad posture reduces oxygen intake, slows circulation, and can compromise the nervous system by starving the brain of vital proprioceptive input. We'll elaborate on the dangers of decreased proprioception later in this chapter.

TEXT NECK SYNDROME

Not just a neck problem

0°	15°	30°	45°	60°
12 lb	27 lb	40 lb	49 lb	60 lb

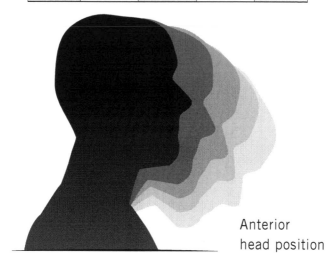

Anterior
head position

A 2017 study in the *International Journal of Medicine* showed that a "highly sedentary life" is a risk factor for *all causes of mortality*.[12] To understand how this looks in modern life, let's look back at Derek, the sedentary worker from the Introduction. We know that he sits for at least eight hours during his workday, and as a result, he has forward head posture. He also sits during his commute to

12 Keith M. Diaz et al, "Patterns of Sedentary Behavior and Mortality in U.S. Middle-Aged and Older Adults: A National Cohort Study," *Annals of Internal Medicine* 167 no. 7 (October 2017). https://doi.org/10.7326/M17-0212.

and from work, while he eats dinner, and when he winds down at the end of the day. We can estimate that he sits for twelve to fourteen hours on a daily basis. Add that to roughly seven hours of sleep, and we're looking at a grand total of twenty-one hours every day with little or no movement.

If movement is essential to life, and Derek is moving only three to four hours each day, I think it's fair to say he's up the creek without a paddle—and his creek will only get more turbulent.

WHAT SHOULD WE DO?

Many of us are a lot like Derek: we know that sufficient exercise is an important factor in both health and longevity, but we fail to move our bodies. Among the obstacles to changing our habits is the overwhelming array of choices at our disposal. Which program(s) should we use? It can be hard to tell, as fitness has exploded into a multi-billion-dollar industry since the mid-1990s, enticing us with the latest and greatest ways to get fit: "Quickly sculpt six-pack abs!" "Burn a thousand calories in thirty minutes!" Everyone tells us that their program is the best, and most of them are indeed beneficial, but how do we know what is truly effective?

Please don't misunderstand us—we are not disparaging exercise programs. Many of them are quite effective, but to experience long-term success, we must be able to incorporate them into our lives. We need to create sustainable, lifelong habits so we don't just aim to lose weight or build muscle, but aim to achieve optimal health. This includes reduced blood pressure, regulated blood sugar, lowered stress levels and risk of heart disease, better joint health, increased energy, and improved mental health and awareness.

Another obstacle is simply the way people perceive their ability (or inability) to move and be active. In our practice, when we encourage patients to exercise, move frequently, and perform a variety of movements throughout the day, we hear responses like, "I'd love to exercise, but I don't feel up to it," or, "I don't have the energy," or, "Once I'm feeling better and the pain goes away, I can be active again."

This feeling, while understandable, is much more related to the patient's perceptions about increasing their activity levels. Frankly, to them, it seems like a lot of pain for little gain. What they often don't realize is how much better general movement and exercise will make them feel, and how it will contribute to their health and well-being— ironically, what they believe to be the problem is actually the solution!

For this reason, we spend time educating our patients

about how movement works in the body. With this knowledge, they can choose movement options that will give them the greatest return on their investment.

THE SCIENCE OF MOVEMENT

Why is movement important? One huge reason is that movement stimulates the nervous system through proprioceptive input to the brain. The cerebellum, which is often referred to as the "little brain," regulates our balance, posture, and coordination. When we move our bodies—particularly the spine—proprioceptors send signals to the cerebellum. Then, the cerebellum sends those signals to the thalamus, and the thalamus in turn relays that information to the cortex where the information is processed and translated into a response within the body. More movement increases proprioceptive signals stimulating the cerebellum, thalamus, and cortex—and more proprioception positively affects our movement, balance, posture, coordination, cognitive ability, and mood.

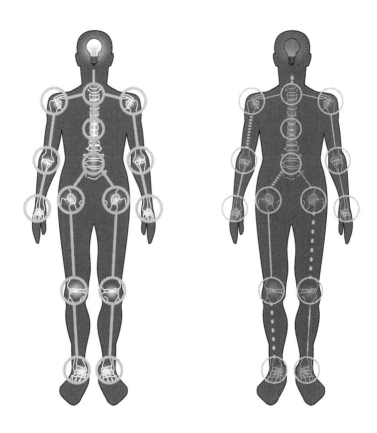

PROPRIOCEPTION

Movement supports proprioception, and proprioception is a part of every movement—it's how the body senses its position in the space around it. During every fraction of every second, the body stimulates the brain with signals, and the brain processes that information. This allows the body to recognize the exact location of every tendon, ligament, joint, and articulation at any given time—we are able to move, react, and respond appropriately to our surroundings.[13]

Proprioception is like our "sixth sense." We usually think of having only five senses—we know we have eyes to see the world, ears to hear our surroundings, tongues to taste the flavors of ice cream and fresh blueberries, our sense of touch to tell us if something is too hot or too cold, and our sense of smell to appreciate the scent of a blooming rose— but proprioception is the superpower sense we didn't learn about in elementary school.

To experience the wonders of proprioception, I invite you to take a moment to do this quick activity: take one hand, extend your index finger, and put it behind your back. Without being able to see, smell, touch, or taste, or hear the location of that finger, take the index finger of your other hand, put it behind your back, and touch the two fingertips together. You're able to do this without any effort, right? That's proprioception.

13   J. C. Rothwell, "Overview of Neurophysiology of Movement Control," *Clinical Neurology and Neurosurgery* 114, no. 5 (June 2012): 432-435. https://doi.org/10.1016/j.clineuro.2011.12.053.

HORMONE PRODUCTION

Movement also stimulates hormone production. *Hormones* are chemical messengers secreted through the endocrine glands, which control and coordinate many functions throughout the body and have a huge influence on our health. Hormones work in response to the level of stress placed upon the body, and that determines if they will work for us or against us. In this section, we'll discuss the hormones that are greatly influenced by and play a role in movement: human growth hormone, catecholamines, and insulin.

Human Growth Hormone (HGH)

Human growth hormone (HGH) is essential for stimulating the growth of almost all tissues in the body. HGH is produced in the pituitary gland, also known as the "Master Gland," which is responsible for sending information from the brain to the glands of the body. It's known for its role in promoting muscle growth and aiding in tissue recovery and repair. HGH also helps to regulate total body composition, and sugar and fat metabolism. Since it's so influential to these functions of the body, it's easy to see why having optimal levels of HGH is crucial to your health and well-being.

There are a few effective ways to stimulate the production of HGH: losing fat, particularly around the midsection; exercising at a high intensity; intermittent fasting; and minimizing sugar intake. In this chapter, we'll focus on the exercise portion.

The main form of physical training in the FIT 5-40-5 program is HIIT, precisely because it has been shown to dramatically stimulate the production of HGH. High HGH helps increase muscle mass and decrease body fat because it competes with insulin on the receptor sites of cells. The presence of HGH can prevent insulin from grabbing glucose as a source of energy. Instead, the body will use stored fat for energy.

With HIIT, you continue to burn fat even during your inactive periods. When coupled with proper nutrition and intermittent fasting, HIIT can help you become a fat-burning machine. It's one of the most effective ways to lose fat quickly, which is great, because fat—belly fat in particular—has been shown to reduce the production of HGH. One study reported that people with three times the average amount of belly fat have up to 50 percent less human growth hormone production than someone without excess fat.[14] If you only have half of your optimal amount of human growth hormone, you significantly hinder your body's ability to keep up with the demands of healing and developing new tissues. Belly fat also puts people at a greater risk for chronic diseases.

DON'T STOP MOVING

Human growth hormone production declines as we age, and this can lead to weight gain, an increase in body fat, fatigue, and lethargy. After retirement, people may not engage in as many activities as they used to, but it's imperative to remain active. We understand there is a tendency to slow down a bit as we age, and slowing down isn't terrible in itself, but movement is an area where there is no room for compromise.

Catecholamines

In addition to boosting levels of HGH, research shows that HIIT is effective in producing *catecholamines*, the hormones more commonly known as *epinephrine* and

---

14   M. Scacchi, A. I. Pincelli, and F. Cavagnini, "Growth Hormone in Obesity," *National Library of Medicine* 23, no. 3 (March 3, 1999): 260-271. https://doi.org/10.1038/sj.ijo.0800807.

norepinephrine. Catecholamines help to mobilize fat stores and increase the level of fat burning.[15]

Here's how it works. Catecholamines are released from the adrenal gland. Intermittent bursts of intense exercise produce much higher levels of catecholamines than moderate exercise, which results in the body burning more fat within the muscles that are being worked, as well as the fat under the skin, such as unwanted belly fat.

When the rate of catecholamines released from the bloodstream increases, breathing rate increases, heart rate speeds up, and blood vessels contract. Blood pressure also rises, increasing blood flow into the large muscles that are used during exercise. Since abdominal and fatty tissue don't typically receive an ample supply of blood or hormones, this increase in circulation helps to mobilize fat, which is then broken down and used as a source of energy.

Epinephrine, more commonly known as *adrenaline*, is the catecholamine that breaks down fat stores and allows them to be used for energy. It also suppresses the appetite, so not only do you burn more fat with high-intensity exercise, you also tend to eat less.

---

15   Leanna M. Ross, Ryan R. Porter, and J. Larry Durstine, "High-Intensity Interval Training (HIIT) for Patients with Chronic Diseases," *National Library of Medicine* 5, no. 2 (June 2016): 139–144. https://doi.org/10.1016/j.jshs.2016.04.005.

HIIT naturally boosts the work of catecholamines and helps to burn fat and suppress appetite, so you can see why the FIT 5-40-5 workout program includes high-intensity workouts.

GET OFF THE TREADMILL

If you spend a lot of time jogging on a treadmill, you may be causing yourself to age faster. You may also be causing joint deterioration and storing fat instead of burning it. This is because longer bouts of cardiovascular exercise (exceeding 50 minutes) decrease testosterone and raise the stress hormone cortisol, so you don't necessarily burn fat. In addition, this type of exercise is an inefficient way to build lean muscle. Also, you might only burn three hundred fifty calories in an hour of jogging, which isn't that much, and you'll probably be hungry soon after. This leads to cravings for sugar-based foods and carbohydrates.

We're not saying that running *won't* help burn calories and keep you lean—we're saying that if you want to mobilize unwanted belly fat or muscular fat, running on a treadmill just won't cut it.

Insulin

Insulin is a hormone produced in the pancreas that regulates blood sugar levels, which are determined by what we eat, and how well our cells respond to the instructions they get from insulin. When you eat, food is broken down and any sugar will circulate through the blood. If blood sugar rises, insulin is released from beta cells in the pancreas. You can think of the process as a messenger system. Insulin binds to a receptor site on the cell and says, "Glucose is here, please let it in."

Insulin Sensitivity and Resistance

Insulin sensitivity is the term used to describe how responsive a person is to the effect of insulin. Generally, the more insulin sensitive you are, the better. When your cells are highly responsive to insulin's message that sugar is available, the sugar is brought into the cell and used as a source of energy, rather than left circulating in the blood.

Conversely, *insulin resistance* occurs when cells don't respond or have a poor response to the presence of insulin. This is a concerning state for the body because if the cells don't recognize the message from insulin, blood sugar levels will remain high.

Let's use an example of arriving at a hotel to illustrate insulin sensitivity and resistance. In this scenario, you arrive at a fancy hotel in a limo. In the case of insulin sensitivity, the driver escorts you to the door and the concierge lets both of you in right away. However, if there is insulin resistance, the concierge may not let you in just yet—he's not responsive to the message from the driver about your arrival.

Now, let's say another guest arrives, and the concierge still doesn't answer. Two more guests arrive, and still no answer. If someone answers the door and lets all of the guests in, the issue is settled. However, if guests continue to arrive and there's no answer, eventually there will be a crowd at the door. In this example, the hotel is a cell, and the guests are glucose. If the guests remain at the "front door" of the cells for too long, they will have elevated levels of blood sugar. If they continue to wait, they get stored as fat, and the problem doesn't end there.

The pancreas will continue to produce insulin, hoping the cells will respond—it sends more information to "turn up the volume," so to speak. The pancreas will encourage the cells to let glucose in by providing more and more insulin. Sometimes that does the trick, and sometimes it doesn't.

More troubling, the pancreas can only do this for so long: if its workload continues to increase, it will eventually reach the point of breakdown. The pancreas is like a student studying for exams—she can do it efficiently for a couple of weeks or so, but if she keeps burning the candle at both ends, she'll end up in a state of burnout. This is also what happens in the body—if the pancreas is overworked, it can result in insulin deficiency, which leads to prediabetes and diabetes.

WHAT IS INSULIN RESISTANCE?

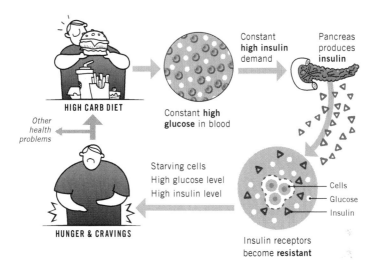

Exercise to the Rescue

Insulin resistance is a big problem, and oftentimes it goes undetected because the symptoms seem benign. Fatigue, weight gain, increased belly fat, sugar cravings, moodiness, fluid retention, and difficulties in concentration and focus don't necessarily indicate that you might be ill; none of these issues are a cause for panic, and we actually consider them to be "normal." Many people think these symptoms are a natural part of aging, but they may be indicators that their health is spiraling out of control.

High-intensity workouts create a high demand for fuel, which helps increase the demand for glucose—the cells will use it as a source of energy. The reduction in blood glucose reduces the demand on the pancreas for insulin production, therefore helping to maintain insulin sensitivity, or even reversing insulin resistance. For people who eat a relatively normal diet and don't have problems with obesity, HIIT can be extremely effective, and it may be all they need to get their desired results.

For people who put too much glucose into their bodies, HIIT is also beneficial, because this type of movement creates a new demand for glucose, making it less likely to be stored as fat. That doesn't give them free rein to eat a lot of sugar, however. Consuming too much sugar isn't good for health in general, so they'd be better off changing their diet along with doing the FIT 5-40-5 workouts. (More on diets in the next chapter.)

For people with increased levels of body fat, HIIT is only partially effective because the demand for glucose will continue. When this is the case, coupling HIIT with intermittent fasting can improve outcomes—the workout alone will yield some results, but combining it with proper nutritional strategies is almost foolproof, and will give health and weight-loss benefits a helping hand.[16]

---

16 Mohammad Asif, "The Prevention and Control the Type-2 Diabetes by Changing Lifestyle and Dietary Pattern," *Journal Education Health Promotion* 3, no. 1 (February 2014). https://dx.doi.org/10.4103%2F2277-9531.127541.

Cortisol

Cortisol is a major stress hormone produced by the adrenal gland, and it plays a significant role in our "fight-or-flight" stress response, weight gain, and weight loss. It's called *cortisol* because of where it's produced: on the cortex of the adrenal glands. At the right levels, it's a useful hormone that helps regulate metabolism, enhances memory and energy, and has an anti-inflammatory effect, along with many other benefits.

However, if cortisol levels remain high for too long, the body believes it's in a crisis and begins to prepare itself for the possibility of starvation—it starts to store more fat on the organs, and the midsection in particular. It's meant to be a protective process if you're really in a crisis, but since you aren't likely to starve, high cortisol doesn't protect you in this scenario; instead, it results in an increase in blood sugar, and your body ends up working against itself.

Cortisol increases with emotional stress, poor diet, pain or chronic pain, inflammation, and a lack of sleep. Cortisol should be at its lowest levels at night, but if you don't get enough good, deep sleep, it can be higher, and that's an issue. People who have higher levels of cortisol may end up with health problems, along with difficulty losing weight. Cortisol also weakens your digestive system, where the majority of your immune cells are housed—and decreased immunity means increased illness.[17]

It's important to note that exercise is a form of stress that temporarily elevates cortisol, but if we exercise regularly, the body will always return to its optimal level of health. Exercise actually *decreases* stress, due to the chemicals it produces. However, the length of intense exercise is important and the FIT 5-40-5 workouts are designed for an ideal duration. Exercising for longer than an hour causes cortisol to circulate through your body for long periods of time. This creates more blood sugar which breaks down in the liver, and you end up with more sugar circulating in your system—this is why exercising for a long duration is not as effective in burning fat.

EFFECTS OF PROLONGED INCREASED LEVELS OF CORTISOL

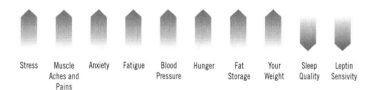

| Stress | Muscle Aches and Pains | Anxiety | Fatigue | Blood Pressure | Hunger | Fat Storage | Your Weight | Sleep Quality | Leptin Sensivity |

MOVING IN 5-40-5 TIME

Now, we would like to introduce you to the Movement component of the FIT 5-40-5 program. This part of the

---

17   Vito Bianchi and Alonzo Esposito, eds., *Cortisol: Physiology, Regulation, and Health Implications* (New York: Nova Science Publishers, 2012).

program consists of high-intensity, short-duration workouts. We do 40-second bursts of 5 different exercises, with a one-minute break following each set. You'll repeat the cycle 5 times. Our core groups of beginner, intermediate, and advanced exercises don't require any weights at all— they are all performed with body weight alone, which gives you the flexibility to exercise anywhere!

All of the workouts involve movement of all four limbs, and we even do the most basic of movements, like jumping jacks. No matter your fitness level, we'll incorporate all four limbs into your exercise program to initiate a greater release of catecholamines, stimulate the production of certain hormones, and inhibit the production of others. That, of course, helps with fat burning both during and after the workout.

At this point, you may be wondering how much movement is necessary to achieve the results you want. Research shows that HIIT can be effective with as little as four minutes of training, but that's mainly for the purpose of decreasing insulin resistance—shorter durations will not produce many of the benefits we've talked about.[18] By working out for longer periods, we get the full benefit of

18   Izumi Tabata et al., "Effects of Moderate-Intensity Endurance and High-Intensity Intermittent Training on Anaerobic Capacity and VO2Max," *Medicine and Science in Sports and Exercise* 28, no. 10 (October 1996). https://doi.org/10.1097/00005768-199610000-00018.

movement, and the body goes through some endurance training, as well.

FITNESS LEVELS

FIT 5-40-5 offers multiple levels of difficulty, modified based on individual goals and needs. Even the beginner level of exercise is effective, because we give sedentary people a realistic and manageable workout, rather than an advanced one—we won't put too much stress on a beginner due to the risk of overexertion or injury. Mechanically speaking, beginner exercises are less stressful on the joints, and more adaptable for people with limitations, such as back pain. As beginners experience fitness improvements, they eventually move to the intermediate level for more of a challenge. This is where the majority of program participants remain.

The advanced level is for people who are established in their athletic pursuits. For example, a British kickboxing champion and a UK award-winning CrossFit coach both went through the advanced course, and they were challenged by each workout. I've found that people who are fit or more athletically inclined push themselves to their limits, because they want a challenge. People in the early stages of their fitness journey may need more encouragement to do the work, but the rule of the FIT 5-40-5 workout is that when you're done, you're *done*. You shouldn't say, "Hey, that was great, I want to do it again!" If you're doing it right and giving it your all, you won't even think about doing another round.

The whole concept of FIT 5-40-5 training is to push yourself. You may not be able to do so the first few times you do it, and beginners might only get through one to three sets. That's normal, and that's okay. The goal is to do the bursts, get the full benefit, and see improvements over time. To ensure you are achieving the right range of heart rate during vigorous activity, we recommend using a heart rate monitor. This will indicate if you are within your target training heart rate range. To find out what this range is for you, it can be calculated using this simple method:

1. Find your max heart rate (MHR) by subtracting your age from 220.
2. For example: 220 – 40 (age) = 180 Max Heart Rate

Next, calculate your resting heart rate (RHR). This is the number of times your heart beats per minute when at rest. I recommend taking this in the morning. Take your pulse and count the number of beats for 10 seconds, then multiply by 6. The result is usually between 60 and 90.

1. Calculate your heart rate reserve (HRR) by subtracting your resting heart rate (RHR) from your maximum heart rate (MHR).

2. For example: 180 − 75 = 105
3. Multiply your HRR by .70 and again by .85 and add your RHR to each number.
4. 105 × .70 = 73.5 + 75 = 148.5
5. 105 × .85 = 89.25 + 75 = 164.25

In this example, your Training Heart Rate (THR) would be between 148.5 and 164.25 beats per minute.

CASE STUDY: DAVID

Before starting FIT 5-40-5, David weighed 24.5 Stone (341 lbs.). He lived a relatively active life until he left high school at the age of eighteen and began working a full-time night shift. Aside from work, his activity levels became virtually non-existent. He admits to making poor food choices regularly. His diet consisted of fast food and he was a frequent visitor of the local pubs. While he knew this wasn't the healthiest lifestyle, he was not fully aware of the overall impact it was having on his health.

The weight piled on, but David continued with this lifestyle. Fast forward to age 39, when David became a father, and he noticed he was unable to even climb a flight of stairs without becoming breathless. He also suffered from chronic low back and knee pain daily.

After visiting his doctor at age 41 to discuss his various health symptoms, his reality was finally delivered to him in no uncertain terms. His doctor told him he wouldn't be around to see his daughter start school if he didn't make a change to his lifestyle—fast!

David's brother referred him to our FIT 5-40-5 program. After a few failed attempts at losing weight and trying to improve his fitness, David considered the program as his last shot at making a change and getting his health under control.

David started the program at 341 lbs. He committed to the system, and after the first 90 days, his weight had dropped by 3 stone, or 42 pounds, and he'd increased his lean muscle mass by 14 percent. Most notable were the eight inches he lost around the waist, reducing dangerous abdominal fat. He reports that he no longer has any back or knee pain and feels better than he has in over twenty years.

Q: How did you feel about the program?

I'm excited about the life ahead. Not only did I get to see my daughter start school, but I'm living a lifestyle that will allow me to see her graduate school and beyond. Another bonus is that I no longer have to shop for clothes in a specialty store designed for larger men."

Q: What was special about FIT 5-40-5?

I was impressed with how well I got on with the meal plan. I am a fussy eater, but it was great to be able to choose my preferences from the Core 40 Food Guide and get healthy and tasty meals every day.

Since completing his FIT 5-40-5 90-Day Transformation, David has continued with FIT 5-40-5. He's lost 88 pounds, and he is nearing his initial goal of losing 100 lbs. For sample workouts in the FIT 5-40-5, 3-Day Challenge, see Appendix G.

CHAPTER 4

////////////

NUTRITION

The food you eat can either be the safest and most powerful form of medicine or the slowest form of poison.

—ANN WIGMORE

Nutritional advice can be overwhelming. It's often difficult to discern the boundary between scientifically accurate advice and popular, trendy diet crazes. At any given time, the "best new program" might offer advice ranging from eating low-fat foods, to cutting carbs, counting calories, only eating at certain times, or limiting yourself to specific foods. The crazy part is that any two approaches may claim they are effective and proven by research, when in fact, they may be completely contradictory.

Diet programs and even reality TV shows teach us the latest, popular ways to eat, but we won't necessarily get a great foundation of nutrients by following a new craze each month. These mixed messages make it seem like the world of nutrition is very complicated, but in reality, it isn't. We are certain that if you had a firm grasp of the basics of nutrition, how the body uses food, and the impact that food has on the body, you would make better choices with relative ease. Ultimately, you could enjoy the benefits of better nutrition, and it would be simple.

RYAN'S STORY

I grew up in a normal" family with two parents, and I had two brothers. We definitely weren't a lazy family. Our father was a rugby coach, so we were introduced to the sport early on, and our holidays to France in our caravan each year involved a lot of outdoor activities. Our eating habits weren't that bad either. My mum fed us what would have been considered a "healthy" diet, following government guidance. We rarely had fizzy drinks, but we did have treats such as biscuits, chocolate, or sweets occasionally.

I was quite a bit bigger than the rest of the kids my age. I struggled to find clothes that fit, having to wear extra-large when most of my friends wore small or medium at most. It made me feel like something wasn't right. I often asked my mum why this was, and she'd reply, "You're just big-boned." I'm not sure if she was protecting me from the truth that I was overweight, or if she really didn't think it was a problem. I knew she was weight-conscious herself, though, since she'd regularly tried different diets or programs to manage her own weight.

My weight became more of an issue as I got older. I began comparing myself to my friends and to other children at my school. I drew attention because of my size and inability to keep up during sports, but I covered this up with an overconfident attitude—I acted as if it didn't matter, taking on the role. I accepted the fact that I was overweight and believed I was just unlucky and got the "fat-genes." Other kids my age ate unhealthy diets and exercised less, but were not my size, so that must've been true; it wasn't in my control to change. For years, I continued to act as if I didn't care about my weight and brushed off comments from others, but after so long, I took them as insults and the overconfidence began to diminish.

Some days I'd return from school with no energy. I was absolutely empty. I felt worthless and broke down in tears, questioning why I was like this. The conclusion was that I was a victim of bad genetics. My mum took me to the doctors, and they confirmed I was clinically obese but couldn't offer me any help as I was too young to go to the gym. They advised a "healthier diet" and more exercise, but it wasn't as if I was eating the wrong things or not exercising in the first place. This left me confused. I felt like no one could help me, but I suppose that was the blessing in disguise. By having no one to save me from my situation, I needed to figure it out myself. I took responsibility, and with that I began to educate myself.

I started doing different forms of exercises and learning how this impacted my fitness. I delved into nutrition, wanting to understand the importance of how it affected my health. And finally, I developed a strong mindset to keep me on track. I learned a lot from my studies, and what

I put into practice has changed and evolved over the years, because science continues to develop and change based on current research. For this reason, I update my knowledge and understanding regularly.

I must say that my transformation wasn't as smooth as it may appear. There were definite highs and lows. It was through my experience as a child feeling helpless, and then learning through the process of change in my own life, that I have decided to continue to learn and share the knowledge required for others to do the same.

IF YOU ONLY KNEW

Before we get into our discussion about nutrition, we need to talk about the importance of water. Water is essential to all bodily functions—it's the most abundant substance in the human body, making up approximately 70 percent of its composition. We *must* drink it regularly, not mixed with anything else—just pure water. And not only is water essential for keeping us hydrated, it serves a role in all systems of the body. It lubricates the joints, helps get rid of waste, regulates our body temperature, helps us to swallow...the list goes on and on.

If we go without water for too long—about three days—our bodies cease to function, and if the absence of water continues for a prolonged period, we will die. It is certainly rare to hear of anyone dying of dehydration in the developed world, since we all know the importance of water, and it's easily accessible.

However, it is true to say that many people experience suboptimal health due to mild dehydration, though the symptoms may not trigger anyone to think that they suffer from a lack of water. For instance, if we were more aware of the connection between water and joint lubrication, we would certainly ensure we had enough water at the first signs of joint pain.

Similarly, if we knew our health could fail in some drastic way due to the absence of specific vitamins or minerals, we most likely wouldn't allow deficiencies to occur. We'd be more likely to reach for a banana if we understood the role of potassium in the body, or more specifically, what happens in the case of potassium deficiency. After all, how many of us suffer from chronic fatigue, muscle cramping, muscle aches, stiffness, weakness, breathing issues, mood changes, or digestive issues? How many people know that these are symptoms of a possible potassium deficiency? Furthermore, who eats a banana as a possible resolution to these problems?

So, just like water, we need an adequate supply of essential vitamins and minerals for proper bodily functions. We need to replenish these through the consumption of quality whole foods on a daily basis if we are to maintain optimal health.

OBSTACLES TO GOOD NUTRITION

Nutrition is simple, but a lot of factors get in the way of its simplicity. A colleague of ours who has seventeen years experience as a dietician with the National Health Service in the UK once told us, "There is a lot of information out there, and much of it is incorrect—people follow flawed advice. Also, many people understand that they need to eat five or more servings of fruits and vegetables every day, but when it comes to nutrition in general, most just leave it to chance."

He went on to say that lack of planning is an obstacle to healthy eating. While there is an abundance of food available to us on demand, the majority of it is unhealthy, processed food. Failure to plan is what often leads us to grab a quick lunch at a fast-food chain at the last minute. As Benjamin Franklin said, "If you fail to plan, you plan to fail."

Now, let's take a closer look at some of the obstacles we face when trying to change our diet for better health.

FOOD QUANTITIES

It's easy to overeat when you consider the typical portion sizes at restaurants today—they are the size of tires on a Monster Truck! People tend to eat more simply because a mass quantity of food is readily available, but much of that food is also processed and purposefully engineered for over-consumption. Never in human history have more foods been readily available to us; we import and export foods all over the globe, and we have developed so many ways of preserving foods to make them last longer. It's no wonder we overeat—food is always right there in front of us!

Many foods today are chemically designed to encourage us to eat more and more—the chemical makeup of these foods bypasses our innate ability to determine that we're full, and that's dangerous. Take potato chips, for example. There's a reason you can't stop until you eat the whole bag. One bag might contain three large potatoes, but your body doesn't seem to get the message that you are overeating.

Unfortunately, many food manufacturers work to get you to eat more without feeling full. It's clever business, but it's the unpleasant and dangerous reality of processed foods.

What's even worse is that "diet" foods that aim to help you reduce weight by eliminating calories that may come from sugar and fat by replacing them with sweeteners, do more harm than good.[19] So, as you can see, overconsumption can be a massive problem, and it can happen when you don't get the message that you are full when eating processed foods. The solution to this problem? Get rid of these "Frankenfoods" that affect the balance between hunger and satiety and wreak havoc on your body's ability to regulate weight. Replace these with real, whole foods, and give your body a chance to get back on track.

SUGAR AND INSULIN

Our bodies are designed to desire foods that appeal to our sense of taste, but unfortunately, what makes certain foods taste good is also what makes them addictive. In fact, sugar and cocaine are similar in how they get you addicted to the substance. A release of hormones associated with the intake of these two keeps you coming back for more, or "get your fix," so to speak.[20]

If you remember our discussion about insulin in the last chapter, consuming too much sugar (which is often hidden in our processed foods) can lead to high blood sugar levels. This leads to the body releasing increased amounts of

---

19 Qing Yang, "Gain Weight by 'Going Diet?' Artificial Sweeteners and the Neurobiology of Sugar Cravings," *Yale Journal of Biology and Medicine* 83, no. 2 (June 2010). https://www.ncbi.nlm.nih.gov/pmc/articles/PMC2892765/.

20 James J. DiNicolantonio, James H. O'Keefe, and William L. Wilson, "Sugar Addiction: Is It Real? A Narrative Review," *British Journal of Sports Medicine* 52, no. 14 (2017). http://dx.doi.org/10.1136/bjsports-2017-097971.

insulin to try and cope with the demands of the excess sugar. If the body is continuously tasked with releasing insulin in an effort to move sugar from the blood into the cells (mainly the liver and muscles), it can result in insulin resistance. The body will begin to secrete more insulin in an effort to use the sugar effectively, and if you're insulin resistant, the sugar can't be brought into the cell to be used for energy. The excess sugar ends up getting stored as fat, which ultimately leads to weight gain.

Leptin

Leptin is another hormone that is a big contributor to weight regulation. It tells us when it's time to eat, and when it's time to *stop* eating. When you feel full and you put down your fork, you can thank leptin for that. However, if you find that you *don't* feel full, it's worth some time and effort to get this hormone in check.

Leptin sends a signal to the brain that we've consumed enough food and our body's energy needs have been met. It also signals the body to increase metabolism and burn the energy that it has, thus balancing energy levels and regulating weight. If the body's leptin feedback loop is working effectively, that means your metabolism is also working well. Brain function should be good, too—your memory is sharp, coordination is solid, and your mood is generally positive.

Just like the other hormones we've discussed, leptin can work effectively for you, or it can work against you. If you have more body fat, you'll make more leptin—your brain receives a signal that you don't need more food or energy, and your metabolism speeds up. If you have less body fat, you'll produce less leptin, and your brain gets a message that the body needs more fuel.

All is well until the wires get crossed. If there's too much leptin going to the receptor, the brain will "tune out" the signals to burn calories and fat, or to increase the metabolic rate. The leptin signal process is like a website: if a site suddenly gets too much traffic, it crashes, and it won't accept any more visitors. Likewise, if there is too much leptin released in the body over a prolonged period, the receptor sites crash and the leptin message won't get through. This is very similar to the problem of prolonged production of insulin. Just as this will result in insulin resistance, a leptin overload can cause weight loss resistance. If you are overweight and tend to overeat, or you are trying to get your weight back in check and you have trouble shifting the pounds, you might have leptin overload.

OBESITY AND THE LEPTIN RESISTANCE CYCLE

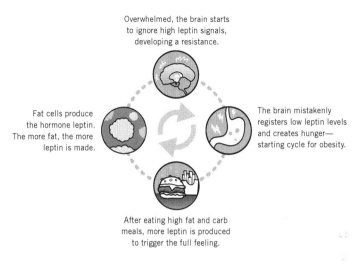

Overwhelmed, the brain starts to ignore high leptin signals, developing a resistance.

Fat cells produce the hormone leptin. The more fat, the more leptin is made.

The brain mistakenly registers low leptin levels and creates hunger—starting cycle for obesity.

After eating high fat and carb meals, more leptin is produced to trigger the full feeling.

Can leptin overload be fixed? You bet! Making proper food choices, like eating from our Core 40 Food Guide (see Appendix B) and engaging in appropriate exercise with the FIT 5-40-5 Fitness Plan, will give your body what it needs to get back in balance and self-regulate.

FAT IS NOT THE ENEMY

More and more people are becoming aware of the health advantages of eating good quality fats, and how they should be an integral part of our diets. However, fat has been demonized for years, and the reasons for this are largely wrong. We're still subject to marketing from an entire industry that is focused on low-fat, fat-free, and "light" foods, with an emphasis on counting calories. We've been taught that as long as you have fewer calories going in than going out, you'll lose weight.

The concept of calorie counting was based on weight gain that was attributed to high-calorie diets. Therefore, to reduce weight, it seemed logical to reduce the calories. If we break macronutrients down to their caloric value, we get 4Kcal for both carbs and proteins, but we get 9Kcal for fat. If this was just a simple numbers game, then it would make the most sense to reduce the nutrient type that yields the most calories: fats. This would work just fine if the body recognized calories, but it doesn't. It recognizes macronutrients.

The body recognizes carbohydrates, proteins, and fats, and it produces a different response when each one is consumed. In short, the body burns and stores fats in response to hormonal instructions. Sugar will spike insulin, fats will not. Therefore, it can be said that sugar is "fattening," while butter is just "fat." The bottom line is, eating good fat does not make you fat!

Another reason fat has a bad rap is because of cholesterol. For many years, health campaigns were certain that the cholesterol from fat—saturated fats in particular—led to heart disease, and therefore we needed to avoid dreaded fats in our diets. This was the birth of the "fat-free" craze, and it was all based on the "lipid hypothesis." The hypothesis states that there is a link between blood cholesterol levels and the occurrence of heart disease. Strangely, they created drugs and were certain of this connection despite the fact it was only ever a hypothesis. Statins, the "wonder drug," came on the scene. These cholesterol-lowering drugs were created to lower blood cholesterol and therefore lower the risk for heart disease. However, with the exception of extremely higher levels of cholesterol, we have yet to see statins significantly reduce the rates of mortality from heart disease. Cholesterol plays several major roles in the body. It is responsible for the creation of hormones, repair of cell membranes, cell protection, and contributes to healthy neurological function, so our constant attempts to lower cholesterol may actually be jeopardizing our health in other ways. The original problem with cholesterol was due to its damaging effects of when it oxidizes and sticks to arterial walls, resulting in a plaque build-up and clogging the arteries.

It is important to remember there are two types of cholesterol: Low Density (LDL) and High Density (HDL). LDL is heavily present in processed fats, which becomes the problem when it is oxidized. However, if we paint all fats with the same brush and listen to convention, we're making a huge mistake. Removing fats from our diet has and will continue to have negative effects on the body. After all, the brain is made up of a significant portion of fat, and depriving the body of fat is just as counterintuitive as depriving it of water. Fortunately, we are well aware of the irreplaceable role fats play in the body and how their consumption is necessary to our well-being. As a result, we have included quality foods that are a great source of fat in our Core 40 Food Guide (see Appendix B) to ensure that you get the health-promoting fats you need.

FOOD QUALITY

We think most people would agree with the statement that food was healthier "back in the day." There is evidence showing that we have to eat eight oranges today to get the same amount of vitamin A that our grandparents would have gotten from one. And it's not just this vitamin we're losing out on: the quantities of protein, calcium, phosphorus, iron, riboflavin (vitamin B2), and vitamin C in common garden crops have all declined over the past half-century. This concept is known as *nutritional inflation*. Our soil is losing nutrient density, predominantly due to high-speed farming—it doesn't have enough time to regenerate and become nutrient dense, and as a result, our food loses mineral quality and quantity.[21]

We also need to consider that food sprayed with chemicals is no longer natural, and the farther away from nature we

---

21 Donald R. Davis, Melvin D. Epp, and Hugh D. Riordan, "Changes in USDA Food Composition Data for 43 Garden Crops, 1950 to 1999," *Journal of the American College of Nutrition* 23, no. 6 (December 2004): 669-682. https://doi.10.1080/07315724.2004.10719409.

get, the closer we get to sickness and disease. It's sad to think that food needs to be labeled "organic," and that it doesn't just come this way as a standard. The unfortunate reality is that in the agricultural process, we use chemicals and make genetic alterations to our food so it isn't affected by insects, pests, and weeds. We make the food unattractive to other living organisms who won't use it as a fuel, but we happily feed it to ourselves. The argument is that the small number of chemicals won't have an effect on our health, but the truth is they have yet to be studied extensively. It's also difficult to isolate what a single factor like pesticides will do to our health over time. The safety stamp of approval is based on incomplete research, and quite possibly very misguided.

More detailed research is in the works to determine the effects of pesticides on our health, but most of us don't need to see the results of a study to conclude that an organic, naturally-grown apple is better than one that was grown with pesticides. Common sense also tells us that regular consumption of a chemical that shouldn't go into the body will eventually lead to harm, one way or another.

Many groups today tout research claiming that genetically modified foods (also known as genetically modified organisms, or GMOs) are safe, when in fact, they are not. Ample research evidence has revealed negative effects of GMOs on our health, but many still debate these findings.[22] [23] We can find research to support both sides of this argument, but when it comes to our health, it is our assertion that we should err on the side of caution.

How Processed Foods Affect the Body

When you come across a label that says "fortified with twelve essential vitamins and minerals" or "packed with healthy grains" or some other lofty claim, put it back on the shelf. The fact is, many of the foods available in grocery stores are processed, loaded with high fructose corn syrup (the worst form of sugar), and pumped full of chemicals that are engineered to increase consumption. It doesn't matter what little nutrients you might get from them—the foods are simply unhealthy and will increase inflammation in the body, a precursor to chronic disease.

Furthermore, the body is not familiar with processed foods. These unnatural foods are often considered to be toxins rather than a usable fuel source. The more processing a food has undergone, the greater the toxic load to the body; and if the body perceives it as a toxin, it must be dealt with as such. The liver will be called into action, indigest-

22 Center for Food Safety, *GE Food & Your Health*. (2020). https://www.centerforfoodsafety.org/issues/311/ge-foods/ge-food-and-your-health.

23 A. S. Bawa and K. R. Anilakumar, "Genetically Modified Foods: Safety, Risks, and Public Concerns—A Review," *Journal of Food Science and Technology* 50, no. 6 (December 19, 2012): 1035–1046. https://dx.doi.org/10.1007%2Fs13197-012-0899-1.

ible "food stuffs" will pass straight through the digestive tract to be excreted, but much of the toxin will get stored in our body's fatty tissue and the toxic effect will remain. Can you see how eating processed foods will contribute to long-term health issues? Rather than being nourishing and contributing to growth and repair, they can leave you malnourished and toxic.

We just expressed that it's essential to have fat in our diets because it plays a crucial role in functions of the body, but it's important to realize how the health benefits can be lost when it's processed. Healthy oils from plant-based sources (avocado, hemp, almond, sesame, etc.) are at potential risk of being damaged through processing. The heat used in processing will oxidize the fats, turning them rancid. This renders them useless by the body, and as a result, they become a toxin. This is why it is best to use cold-pressed oils.

It's also important to avoid fats that have been hydrogenated to help increase their stability and the shelf life of the foods they are in. This processing may help the food last longer and keep it looking pretty, but it will have the opposite effect on your life expectancy. Our advice is to stay well clear of these fats, which is easy to do when you consume a diet made up of whole, natural foods.

DEFINING A HEALTHY DIET

So, what should you eat? While no one diet is perfect for everyone, there is one that is perfect for *you*. The word "diet" is confusing, because it can describe an intentional way of eating (gluten-free, for example), or it can simply define food consumption habits in general. The key is to not let your diet become a *diet*. You shouldn't stress about which diet to choose, or how to eat—the focus should be on *what* you eat.

Versatility is important when it comes to eating, and stringent meal plans are difficult to maintain—determining your diet is an ever-evolving, personal process. For example, eating three square meals a day can be effective if you want to maintain your current weight, but eating five small meals a day will work better if you want to boost your metabolism. There are different ways to eat, and your goals, along with how you want to feel, will ultimately determine the pattern you choose.

VITAMINS AND MINERALS

The best diets place emphasis on eating the proper amounts of fruits and vegetables because they naturally contain most of the vitamins and minerals that we need. Vitamins are essential to many processes of the body, fuel enzyme activity, and serve as antioxidants and cofactors.

For example, vitamin B12 acts as a coenzyme in the body's cell metabolism, contributes to the production of DNA, and metabolizes fatty and amino acids. It is literally crucial to our survival. Vitamin C, E, and beta-carotene are vitamins that serve as antioxidants. They can donate a hydrogen atom and neutralize a free radical, reducing oxidative stress in the body and lowering your risk of many chronic diseases.

Adequate mineral intake is equally important, but the benefits of minerals are not as commonly known. They contribute to the formation of bones and teeth, but they also play a much more significant role: they are required for normal nerve function. And since the nervous system controls everything in the body, a mineral deficiency can have serious negative consequences.

Through copious amounts of research and testing, we can determine how much of a particular vitamin or mineral we should consume. Through different stages of life—such as pregnancy, or during other physiological changes—we may require more of certain vitamins and minerals than others, and government-determined recommendations can help us make the right choices. Despite these sound recommendations and the fact that research reveals that detrimental things happen to the body in the absence of vitamins and minerals, some of us still continue a diet with minimal nutrient content.

If you are eating adequate amounts of fruits and vege-tables, we commend you for a job well done. However, if you aren't, then it's likely that you're deficient in key vitamins, minerals, and nutrients. You have to make a change. For some, this is difficult and it is acceptable to supplement your food intake with quality supplements. This is better than going without. In Appendix C, we have added a list of recommended supplements we advise for many clients.

FATTY ACIDS

Omega-3 fatty acids cannot be produced by the body on its own, and must be obtained from your diet. There are three main types: eicosapentaenoic acid (EPA), docosahexae-noic acid (DHA), and alpha-linolenic acid (ALA). EPA and DHA are easiest for the body to absorb and utilize from food. ALA is converted from EPA and DHA in the body so it can be used and is primarily found in plant-based sources. For this reason, it is often said that vegans who do not eat animal sources of omega-3 may develop a deficiency. Omega-3 is important because it has a role in nearly every aspect of your health, one of the most import-ant being decreasing inflammation.[24]

The optimal ratio between omega-6 and omega-3 fatty

---

24   Juan Garrido-Maraver et al., "Coenzyme Q10 Therapy," *Molecular Syndromology* 5, nos 3–4 (July 2014): 187–197. https://doi.org/10.1159/000360101.

acids is four to one. This can be very difficult to attain, as many foods today are much higher in omega-6. A lot of animals are fed corn and soy, therefore making their meat high in omega-6 also. When an animal is fed an unnatural diet—for example, a cow being fed grains when it should be grazing on grass—this leads to an imbalance in their bodies. They then become susceptible to sickness and disease, and the animal may require interventions to keep them alive. This disease is then passed down the food chain when we consume these animals, leading to a bodily state of inflammation, rather than decreasing it if we were to have more omega-3 (as intended).

To give another example of this skewed ratio, fish used to be a great source of omega-3, but this is no longer the case. Commercially available fish are often farmed, which means they are fed pellets instead of their natural diets and given hormones in a bid to keep them from getting sick. This disrupts the ratio of omega-6 and omega-3, and most farm-fed fish contain too much omega-6. The best option for humans to obtain high omega-3 is to eat wild fish—the ones that eat a natural diet in a natural habitat.

To combat these distorted ratios, supplementing with omega-3 can help, but choosing animal products that have consumed natural diets will prevent ratio balance from becoming an issue.

Other Important Vitamins

Since certain natural foods like meat and fish no longer carry the rich nutrients that we require, it raises a strong argument for quality nutritional supplementation to some degree. Our recommendations can be found in Appendix C. Here, we will emphasize some key vitamins and minerals.

CoQ10

Coenzyme Q10 is an essential element for many daily functions and is required by every single cell in the body. Oxidation of cells is one of the main contributors to aging, and CoQ10 serves as an antioxidant in the body to prevent (oxidation). This essential nutrient is known as the "powerhouse of the cell" and is involved in energy production. Tiny, specialized cells called *mitochondria* turn nutrients into usable sources of energy and CoQ10 that is required during this process.

CoQ10 is well absorbed by the body, and quality fatty fish, spinach, cauliflower, and broccoli contain this nutrient. Alternatively, supplementing is equally effective, especially if taken along with food, and can contribute to maintaining good levels in your body.[25] CoQ10 is especially important for maintaining a healthy heart and is believed

---

25 Juan Garrido-Maraver et al., "Coenzyme Q10 Therapy," *Molecular Syndromology* 5, nos. 3–4 (July 2014): 187–197. https://doi.org/10.1159/000360101.

to be associated with conditions such as diabetes, cancer, fibromyalgia, heart disease, and cognitive decline.[26]

Magnesium

Magnesium is another mineral that plays a significant role in the human body. It resides in our cells, so blood tests generally don't indicate if we're deficient or not. For this reason, your doctor may not pay much attention to it. However, magnesium calms muscles, including the heart, the nerves, and the brain; and when magnesium levels are too low, muscles can become twitchy.

Magnesium is found in meat but can be lost in the cooking process. It is also found in high quantities in dark green vegetables but can also be lost in the cooking process. A supplement for magnesium can be a good option to counteract the effects of not getting enough through diet alone.

Vitamin D

Vitamin D is critical for bone density, a healthy immune system, and sufficient production of testosterone. Unlike the other nutrients we've described, it doesn't come from food. Vitamin D is particularly important for those who don't live in sunny environments, since a primary source of the vitamin comes from direct exposure to sunlight. Vita-

---

26   Ibid.

min D3 is the particular type of product for those looking to supplement their vitamin D levels, as it cuts out the middleman and doesn't require absorption, breakdown, or conversion by the body—it gives the body exactly what it needs.

Go Big on Greens

Finally, and probably one of our top recommendations to ensure you get enough vitamins and minerals is with a greens powder. These are becoming ever more popular as a "go-to" supplement to ensure that you get a whole host of valuable nutrients in an easy way. The process by which the nutrients from plants can be condensed and extracted has become more advanced and is increasingly able to keep the vitamins, minerals, and antioxidants intact. Provided it contains a wide variety of quality organic ingredients, the greens powder can be a great way to augment a healthy diet.

In addition, if the food you eat doesn't provide enough of the nutrients discussed in this section, we strongly advise that you include a quality greens powder and multivitamin/mineral or a vitamin- and mineral-rich meal replacement in your daily routine.

We created the nutritional component of FIT 5-40-5 based on the basic understanding of food, vitamins, minerals, and recommended daily intakes discussed in this chapter. We've selected 40 nutrient-dense foods and divided them into groups to create what is known as the "Core 40 Food Guide"—and we want our foods to help the body work properly and maximize its ability to express health. (See the Core 40 Food Guide in Appendix B.)

The key takeaway here is simple: if you want to be healthy, then eat a variety of real foods and supplement when necessary. Choose as many foods as possible that have a single ingredient, so you can be confident they haven't been processed. Any time you substitute any whole foods—such as good quality meats, vegetables, seeds, or nuts—with a processed version, you increase your risk of sickness, disease, and overall poor health.

POPULAR DIETS

To help inform your choice of diet, we'll cover the benefits and pitfalls of a few common ones in this section. We don't take a particular stance on any of them—we're simply highlighting their strengths and identifying pitfalls and points of caution. You can make your own decision based on this information and your personal preferences.

PALEO DIET

The Paleo diet was inspired by the way our Paleolithic

hunter-gatherer ancestors ate, and it encourages us to eat the way we were "designed" to eat. Health experts consider it to be one of the healthiest diets—it helps us to stay lean and maintain energy levels and strength. The emphasis on eating high-quality, organic foods minimizes chemical stress on the body. The Paleo diet consists of a variety of proteins from various animal sources, including fatty cuts of meat and runny eggs—cooking is done in such a way that the fats are left intact. Organ meats are also part of this diet. Traditional diets often push these cheap cuts of meat to the side, but Paleolithic man would never have let these nutrient-dense morsels go to waste.

Vegetables are also a huge part of the diet along with nuts and seeds. Eating Paleo provides a phenomenal number of antioxidants, vitamins, minerals, and vital nutrients from these natural foods, which are crucially important to our health and wellness. They are also associated with a decrease in chronic disease.[27]

Fats are included in the Paleo diet as well, with avocados and olive oil being two common sources. These choices are popular because they taste good, are great sources of fat, and can be used in a variety of ways.

---

27 Heiner Boeing et al., "Critical Review: Vegetables and Fruit in the Prevention of Chronic Diseases," *European Journal of Nutrition* 51, no. 6 (September 2012): 637–663. https://dx.doi.org/10.1007%2Fs00394-012-0380-y.

Potential Pitfalls

The intent of the Paleo diet is for people to consume grass-fed, naturally-raised beef that is high in Omega-6s, and free of antibiotics and hormones. However, the quality of meat can be a pitfall with this diet. If the source is not responsibly raised, the meat is pro-inflammatory, and eating it defeats the purpose of the diet.

Another pitfall of this diet is the quantity of meat consumed. This diet recommends that you consume far more meat than our Paleolithic ancestors did—and red meat, in particular, is associated with an increased risk of heart disease and cancer.[28]

Despite these potential pitfalls, Paleo diets are typically rich in Omega-3 fats, which can dramatically reduce instances of obesity and contribute to the reduction of cancer, diabetes, and neurological decline.

VEGETARIANISM

The Vegetarian Society defines a vegetarian as "someone who lives on a diet of grains, pulses, legumes, nuts, seeds, vegetables, fruits, fungi, algae, yeast and/or some other non-animal-based foods (e.g., salt) with, or without, dairy

---

28 Yan Zheng et al., "Association of Changes in Red Meat Consumption with Total and Cause Specific Mortality among US Women and Men: Two Prospective Cohort Studies," *The BMJ* 365 (June 12, 2019): l2110. https://dx.doi.org/10.1136%2Fbmj.l2110.

products, honey and/or eggs. A vegetarian does not eat foods that consist of or have been produced with the aid of products consisting of or created from any part of the body of a living or dead animal. This includes meat, poultry, fish, shellfish, insects, byproducts of slaughter, or any food made with processing aids created from these."[29]

Since vegetarians eat a plant-based diet, they almost always get adequate vitamins and minerals from the foods they eat. They also get more nutrients from their food than vegans, since they eat animal byproducts like eggs, dairy, and other sources of fat, while vegans don't consume any animal products.

Vegetarians consume vital nutrients that play a role in cancer prevention, and they don't run the risk of eating too much meat. They also take in plenty of dietary fiber, magnesium, folic acid, vitamin C, and iron.

Potential Pitfalls

A potential pitfall of the vegetarian diet is that it can be difficult to balance Omega-6s and Omega-3s. It's also possible to create a B12 deficiency because only small amounts of this vitamin are found in eggs and dairy. A vegetarian can get B12 from another source, such as yogurt, but they

---

29   The Vegetarian Society, "What Is a Vegetarian?" (2020). https://vegsoc.org/info-hub/definition/.

most likely won't consume enough to get the necessary amount.

Another potential pitfall is the possibility of eating too many carbohydrates. If vegetarians eat a lot of bread, for example, they're consuming refined carbohydrates in excess, which will ultimately become sugars when they're broken down.

Despite these pitfalls, vegetable-based diets are usually lower in calories, and can be beneficial for people with issues such as diabetes and obesity.

VEGANS AND NUTRIENT DEFICIENCIES

Vegans follow a vegetarian diet but take things a step further: they avoid all animal products such as dairy, eggs and honey, leaving them with a predominantly plant-based diet. Reasons can vary as to why someone chooses to follow a vegan diet, but it can typically result in better health, increased weight loss, and protection against chronic diseases. The majority of the positive health effects of this diet may be attributed to the reduction of meat and dairy consumption, and the increase in consumption of plant-based foods.

Potential Pitfalls

One of the most common things you'll likely hear about a

vegan diet is that it lacks protein, because the type of protein found in plants does not always contain the complete amino acid profile required for growth and repair. However, a conscious vegan can eat from a variety of plants or plant-based protein sources to give them a complete profile of proteins. Similar to vegetarian diets, vitamin B12, iron, zinc, and omega-3 fatty acids should be carefully monitored to avoid the negative health effects that can occur by not consuming enough of these nutrients.

As previously mentioned, vegans may suffer reduced levels of DHA, a type of Omega 3, due to its difficulty being converted in the body from plant sources, and this can lead to health implications, such as reduced brain function.[30] [31]

Finally, due to the rise in popularity of this diet, there has been an increase in the promotion of vegan products and the introduction of meat substitutes. For example, sausages and burgers are made with plant-based protein sources, such as pea or soy protein.

Quality always needs to be considered when buying these foods, and not all vegan-friendly foods are healthy. They

---

30 Theresa Greupner et al., "Effects of a 12-Week High-A-Linolenic Acid Intervention on EPA and DHA Concentrations in Red Blood Cells and Plasma Oxylipin Pattern in Subjects with a Low EPA and DHA Status," *Food and Funcion* 9, no. 3 (March 2018). https://doi.org/10.1039/c7fo01809f.

31 Anthony F. Domenichiello, Alex P. Kitson, and Richard P. Bazinet, "Is Docosahexaenoic Acid Synthesis from A-Linolenic Acid Sufficient to Supply the Adult Brain?" *Progress in Lipid Research* 59 (July 2015): 54-66. https://doi.org/10.1016/j.plipres.2015.04.002.

can still be pumped full of added sugar, preservatives, and trans fats, which are not advised in a healthy lifestyle.

KETOGENIC DIET

A ketogenic diet consists of high-fat and moderate protein consumption, with low or no carbohydrate intake. The standard ratio is 75/20/5 percent. The body uses different energy sources, and in the absence of carbohydrates, it will begin to use fat as a primary source of fuel, which is known as *nutritional ketosis*. Benefits of ketosis include weight loss and a decrease in body fat. It has also been shown to help regulate blood sugar levels and improve the sensitivity of hormones such as leptin and insulin. It has also been shown to improve heart health, slow cancer growth, and reduce inflammation and the severity of epilepsy and seizure disorders. There are a whole host of benefits when it is done correctly.[32]

Potential Pitfalls

The attractive lure of eating high-fat foods can often put people on a path to eating fatty foods instead of focusing on healthy ones. Consistently eating conventional meats that are high in toxins may lead to a loss of body fat, but it can also lead to an accumulation of toxins within the body and a decrease in health. Due to carbohydrates, there may

32 Jennifer T. Batch et al., "Advantages and Disadvantages of the Ketogenic Diet: A Review Article," *Cureus* 12, no. 8 (August 2020). https://doi.org/10.7759/cureus.9639.

be a lack of fruit and vegetable consumption, which introduces the problem of vitamin and mineral deficiency. Close attention must be paid to choosing healthy fat sources and good quality meat when following a ketogenic diet.

INTERMITTENT FASTING

Intermittent fasting (IF) is not necessarily a diet—it's more of a method or practice that you can *incorporate* into your diet. Intermittent fasting is effective because it forces the body to use its entire stores of carbohydrates as fuel. Once those are all gone, it dips into fat as its primary source of energy. Intermittent fasting is a good way to mobilize and burn fat that is being stored unnecessarily.

So where does our energy come from while we aren't eating? Toward the end of a fast, your body goes into *ketosis,* where it will burn ketones for energy. Ketones are produced when the body must burn fat for fuel and are derived from the mitochondria of liver cells that break down fatty acids. We used to believe that glucose was the best source of energy, but over the years we've discovered that our bodies can also use fat efficiently. Once people adjust to fasting, their blood sugar regulates, they have higher energy levels, and experience sharper mental acuity.[33]

---

33 Valter D. Longo and Satchidanada Panda, "Fasting Circadian Rhythms, and Time Restricted Feeding in Healthy Lifespan," *Cell Metabolism* 23, no. 6 (June 14, 2020): 1048–1059. https://dx.doi.org/10.1016%2Fj.cmet.2016.06.001.

THE THREE-DAY FAST

As mentioned in Chapter 3, coupling IF with HIIT is an effective way to burn fat and reverse insulin resistance. However, it is not appropriate for everyone. For some, getting their metabolism working effectively is the first priority, so eating regularly will help them accomplish this.

Intermittent fasting is most suitable for those who want to recover from illness, want to improve the function of their nervous system, or need to lose a considerable amount of weight. If this is you, a three-day fast might be appropriate to kick-start the process of nutritional ketosis before you begin intermittent fasting.

The lengthier fast rapidly uses up glucose reserves in the body. Then, the body must break down fatty acids for energy, which results in the production of ketones in the liver. The body then begins to slow growth signaling and increases its resistance to cellular stress. Prolonged fasting has also shown promising results for immunity, inflammation, neurogenesis, and metabolic health. These benefits may be associated with lower-level hormones such as IGF-1 and insulin. While it may sound like not eating for this long can be damaging, it is really the opposite. Fasting boosts levels of beneficial hormones, specifically human growth hormone (HGH), and helps to boost the body's natural ability to heal itself.[34]

---

34   V. D. Longo and M. P. Mattson, "Fasting: Molecular Mechanisms and Clinical Applications," *Cell Metabolism* 19, no. 2 (February 2014): 181-92. https://dx.doi.org/10.1016%2Fj.cmet.2013.12.008.

FIT 5-40-5 NUTRITION DONE RIGHT

The standard nutritional practice of the FIT 5-40-5 program is to eat five times a day: either two meals and three snacks, or three meals and two snacks, depending upon individual goals and needs. The "Core 40 Food Guide" separates foods into five categories, with eight foods in each one. We recommend that participants eat five different foods from the Core 40 each day. The included list of foods is not an exhaustive one, but using it as a guide will help ensure that your body receives the proper variety of nutrients on a daily basis.

The foods recommended in this program are rich in antioxidants to increase energy and help combat oxidative stress. We emphasize diverse, well-rounded diets, strongly promote single-ingredient foods, and encourage participants to stay away from processed or refined foods. We also ask participants to avoid foods that are high on the glycemic index (the ones that tend to spike blood sugar), or carbs that don't add valuable nutrients to the diet.

THE GLYCEMIC INDEX

When we eat food, our body will aim to convert this into energy so that it can be used in the body. For most carbohydrates, this means turning them into glucose or blood sugar. Not all foods will digest at the same speed or to the same extent.

The scale typically runs from 0-100, the higher the number the quicker and bigger the effect on blood sugar and the insulin response. Foods like bread, pasta, and rice tend to be high up on the scale; and broccoli, cauliflower, and cabbage will be lower.

When you're trying to achieve your health goals, whether that is to lose excess body fat, or improve your hormonal health for energy and mood, taking into account the glycemic index of foods is extremely important, as every spike in blood sugar requires an insulin response to stabilize it.

GENERAL RECOMMENDATIONS

We recommend that you stick to the Core 40 Food Guide most of the time, but following the FIT 5-40-5 nutrition plan is not as daunting as it might appear—there is room for flexibility. The plan does have "non-negotiables," such as vegetables, but we know that restrictive meal plans result in failure, so we don't ask you to be rigid with your eating. If you want to sweeten something with honey, that's fine. Or, if you're out with your kids on a hot summer day and want to have ice cream, then by all means, treat yourself. Just don't take advantage of the flexibility, and don't eat processed foods on a regular basis.

There are many foods that can deliver great health benefits, but they shouldn't become staples in your diet—these are "negotiables," and they are allowed in small amounts. Greek yogurt, for example, is good for you, but it may not be the best source of nutrients. If you have some with breakfast every day, that's not going to cancel out all of your efforts. Eating Greek yogurt does have its benefits, but some people can't tolerate eating dairy very often.

Our personal philosophies about health are important, but we have to acknowledge that sometimes they can lead us down the wrong path. Our best advice is to use common sense when making decisions about your diet, and if something isn't working well, change it. This can be difficult when we've been hard-wired to think in certain ways, but your health is definitely worth the effort! (See Appendix G for a 3-Day FIT 5-40-5 Sample Meal Plan.)

CASE STUDY: KIERAN

Kieran started the FIT 5-40-5 program at age 25 and weighed 282 lbs. He was a keen soccer player in his teen years and lived a healthy and active lifestyle. However, this changed when his grandmother passed away. He became somewhat of a recluse. He didn't leave his house often, and his social life was no longer on the soccer field. Rather, he spent endless hours online, sitting in front of a computer and gaming. Kieran continued with this lifestyle until he was age 25, when his older brother tragically passed away in his sleep.

By this time, Kieran was obese, and inactivity and a poor diet perpetuated his situation. Motivated by the loss of his brother and his mother's fear for his health, Kieran started the FIT 5-40-5 program.

Kieran felt the program might be too much for him at first, or that maybe he had let himself go too far and now exercise was beyond him. He also suffered from chronic low back pain, which he believed would be a hindrance in his ability to make a change.

During his first 5-40-5 workout, Kieran could only manage two sets before he was unable to continue. However, within two weeks, he was able to complete the full 5 sets.

Kieran was surprised at how well he managed to perform the workouts and made a commitment to see the program through with complete effort in all three areas: exercise, nutrition, and mindfulness.

Kieran weighed 282 lbs. when he started the program. Over the course of 90 days, he lost 37 lbs. and seven inches off his waistline.

Q: What did you like about the Fit 5-40-5 program?

I was inspired by the large improvement in my weight, fitness level, and strength in such a short period of time. I started feeling like my former self, and it brought me a huge sense of satisfaction to be feeling so much better. I am back to living a more fulfilled life and enjoying every day. I lost my way for a while, but I feel back in control of my destiny. The FIT 5-40-5 program has done more for me than I can explain.

Q: What was special about the FIT 5-40-5 program?

I love the overall simplicity. I love how the daily program was delivered; it was so easy to follow. What helped me most, particularly in the first month, was having online coaching support in the close community. The daily support was exactly what I needed to keep me on track.

Kieran has continued with the FIT 5-40-5 program. To date, he's gone from a shirt size of XXXL to an L, and has lost 87 pounds, bringing him under the 200-pound mark for the first time in seven years.

CHAPTER 5

////////////

THE MIND

The mind is a powerful force. It can enslave us or empower us. It can plunge us into the depth of misery or take us to the heights of ecstasy. Learn to use the power wisely.

—David Cuschieri

We believe the essence of who we are is the result of the experiences we've had throughout our lives. These experiences have established the way we perceive the world and the way we see ourselves in it. Take a moment to think about who you are. How do you view the world? How was this version of you created?

We often view the world in black and white. We see the possible and impossible, can- and can't-dos, rights and wrongs, and shoulds and should-nots. To that end, the way we perceive reality ultimately dictates who we are and conditions how we live. If we want to create a different version of ourselves, we have to initiate change.

For example, if you want to transform from a couch potato to a fit athlete, it is no secret that you can't continue with your current unhealthy behaviors and beliefs—you have to ditch the chips and Twinkies and begin to prioritize exercise and nutrition. The older you are and the longer you've held on to certain beliefs, the harder it is to "rewire" your brain. If you truly want to change, you have to create a new, dominant state of being. In other words, you have to rewire your mind. In this chapter, we will share an overview on how to get started doing exactly that.

A LOOK INSIDE THE BRAIN

In order to understand how to begin rewiring your mind, we must start by discussing the brain. The studies surrounding the brain are expansive and exciting, and we still have much to learn about it. We don't know as much about the brain as we do about the science of nutrition and movement, but fortunately, our current level of understanding is adequate—we have enough information about how to influence changes in the brain and effectively create transformation. The structure and function of the brain are far from simple, but for the sake of simplicity, we've divided its functions into three parts: Thinking, Doing, and Being.

THINKING

The outer surface (or the first level) of the brain is the *neo-cortex*—it takes in and analyzes information and controls our conscious thoughts. The neocortex plays a key role in understanding the process of change, and it influences how you act based on what you learn. It also responds to new stimuli and allows for reasoning and rationale. This is the largest area of the brain, controlling language, consciousness, spatial awareness, motor commands, and sensory perception. It has only been since the turn of the twenty-first century that scientists have discovered that the adult neocortex can generate new neurons in a process known as *neurogenesis*.[35] This new understanding allows for the possibility of retraining adult brains and reinforcing new connections. Simply put, you are not "stuck" in your current state of being. If you want to create newer, healthier habits, then your brain is specifically built to help you do exactly that.

DOING

The next level of the brain is known as the *limbic system*, a group of structures which include the amygdala, hippocampus, and the thalamus. These structures are responsible for your feelings, which in turn are derived from mood, memory, and hormone control. The amygdala houses our

---

35 Fred H. Gage, "Neurogenesis in the Adult Brain," *Journal of Neuroscience* 22, no. 3 (February 2002): 612-613. https://doi.org/10.1523/JNEUROSCI.22-03-00612.2002.

emotions, and the hippocampus processes information during learning. This is also where we process new experiences from emotional memories. The thalamus integrates all incoming sensory information to various parts of the conscious thinking brain.[36] Since this area of the brain helps regulate endocrine function in response to emotional stimulus, it becomes crucially important to control our emotional input in order to help achieve optimal health.

BEING

The third level of the brain is the *cerebellum*—this is the memory center. The memories created in the limbic brain are stored here. For this reason, it's also been said that the cerebellum is home to our personality. Its other roles include coordinating movement and balance and facilitating hardwired memories and behaviors. Interestingly, the cerebellum makes up roughly 10 percent of the brain's mass, but it houses more than 50 percent of its total neurons, making it the most active area of the brain.[37] So not only is the cerebellum crucial in contributing to our body's physical capabilities, it is also crucial to our cognitive processing and emotional control.[38] We will see how emotions impact our

---

36 D. M. Katz and K. Chandar, *Encyclopedia of the Neurological Sciences*, 2nd ed. (2014): 425–430.

37 D. M. Katz and K. Chandar, *Encyclopedia of the Neurological Sciences*, 2nd ed. (2014): 643–650.

38 Mark Rapoport, Robert van Reekum, and Helen Mayberg, "The Role of the Cerebellum in Cognition and Behavior," *The Journal of Neuropsychiatry* 12, no. 2 (May 2000). https://doi.org/10.1176/jnp.12.2.193.

health in this chapter which will highlight the important role the cerebellum plays in the health of our mind and body.

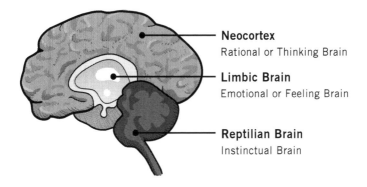

Neocortex
Rational or Thinking Brain

Limbic Brain
Emotional or Feeling Brain

Reptilian Brain
Instinctual Brain

THE PROCESS OF CHANGE

If we want to change our being, we must think, feel, and act differently than we currently do. If we continue with the same experiences, we often have the same thoughts, actions, and behaviors as a result. Essentially, we continue to be the same. The repetition of thoughts and feelings results in the persistence of our current reality. However, we can change our brain through "mental rehearsal," where we change the way we think about a familiar event—we can elicit different actions and behaviors in response to new thoughts.[39] Doing this repeatedly over time can rewire the brain and help us create a new reality.

---

39 D. Pascual-Leone et al., "Modulation of Muscle Responses Evoked by Transcranial Magnetic Stimulation During the Acquisition of New Fine Motor Skills," *Journal of Neurophysiology* 74, no. 3 (1995): 1037–1045.

Another possible way to create change is through the introduction of new information, followed by hands-on experience and instruction using this new knowledge. You pay attention to the experience you're learning, absorb the new action, and then repeat the experience until it becomes a new behavior. As you apply what you've learned and move through the new experience, you create new patterns to replace the old. You will literally change your brain, or your state of "being."

When you begin to have new experiences and create new thought patterns, the limbic brain produces chemicals that connect the mind and body.[40] When this process happens repeatedly, the new patterns continue to get stronger until they are imprinted into the subconscious. For example, think of when you learned to ride a bike. If you can remember that experience, it started with you wanting to learn to ride, and getting instructions on how to perform the new activity possibly from a parent or older sibling. This was followed by the physical experience, which was a bit difficult at first. You tried to put all of the actions together: you steadied the handlebars, kept the pedals moving, watched for obstacles, etc.

Eventually, through repetition, the process of riding a bike became second nature. You didn't need to think about

---

40   Candance B. Pert, *Molecules of Emotion: Why You Feel the Way You Feel* (New York: Scribner, 1997).

what to do; you simply jumped on the bike and off you went, working on autopilot from the subconscious. The skill of how to ride your bike became hardwired in your brain.

If we keep the same thoughts, actions, and feelings, we can't change—if we don't let them go, we will only perpetuate the same version of ourselves. By consciously introducing new information and changing the way we think, we can embrace new actions and facilitate real change. For example, if you decided to adopt the Paleo diet, you'd have to learn which foods to prioritize, to create new meal plans, and to begin eating in a new way. Then, you'd repeat this new behavior over and over again. By doing this, the previous hardwiring to eat lots of carbs and sweets would eventually be replaced by new behaviors, and healthier eating would become the new norm.

People who are always willing to try new things, go new places, and embrace new experiences may find it easy to create change. Those who don't might find it more difficult. For some, even the *thought* of making a change breeds feelings of insecurity, anxiety, and fear. For example, a person who is inactive and uncomfortable with their body image might get overly anxious about going to the gym. Those feelings are understandable, but ultimately counterproductive. Staying in your comfort zone is the antithesis of change.

Furthermore, our addiction to our current life can be so strong that it sabotages our attempts to change. Many people feel compelled to stay in a place that is less than ideal, or even in a place of misery, because at least they know what to expect there—they'd rather stick with the familiarity of unhappiness than take a risk due to fear of the unknown.

HOOKED ON A FEELING

Most of the time, we associate being "hooked" with an addiction to drugs, alcohol, or sugary foods—it's rare for us to think of emotional addiction, though the phenomenon is at least as common, and very real.[41] When I say, "addicted to the familiar," it's not a metaphor; we really can get "Hooked on a Feeling." (I don't know if B. J. Thomas was aware of the science surrounding the lyrics of his classic song, but he certainly got it right.)

Emotional addiction is caused by a chemical reaction in the brain that occurs in response to the production and release of *neuropeptides*, which influence cells within the brain and body—they facilitate communication between groups of neurons.[42] For example, let's say a particular event or recurring circumstance in your life elicits feel-

---

41   Robert Plutchik, *Emotions and Life: Perspectives from Psychology, Biology, and Evolution* (Washington, D.C.: American Psychological Association, 2002).

42   Arthur C. Guyton, *Textbook of Medical Physiology* (San Diego: Harcourt Publishing, 1990).

ings of anger. This creates increased levels of stress and releases stress hormones which give the body a rush of energy. Your brain will release neuropeptides through the bloodstream, and they will bind to receptor sites for the chemical released in response to "anger" throughout the body.

It works the same way with drug addiction: the more frequently a drug is ingested, the more it will bind to receptor sites. With increased use of heroin, for instance, the body creates more receptor sites that yearn for heroin neuropeptides, and the cells demand more of the drug.[43] If the addict stopped ingesting heroin, the cells would send strong signals to the brain begging for more.

This process also holds true when it comes to our emotions. Although our body is designed to deal with stress for a short duration and then return to balance, if a person continually feels anger in response to external events or stimuli, it wears down the related receptor sites, while sparking the production of new sites that demand more of the chemical released from the feeling of anger.

This physical reaction could be the result of long-term repression, verbal abuse, feelings of low self-worth, or

---

43   Alan D. Kaye et al., "Prescription Opioid Abuse in Chronic Pain: An Updated Review of Opioid Abuse Predictors and Strategies to Curb Opioid Abuse," *Pain Physician* 20, no. 2S (February 2017): S93-S109. https://pubmed.ncbi.nlm.nih.gov/28226333/.

even a daily circumstance. If a person feels anger for long enough, they can enter a cycle of emotional addiction—they unconsciously seek out more anger, often from a familiar situation because it's the easiest way to meet the body's demand for the chemical. This is why some people stay in undesirable situations—they are literally "hooked on a feeling."

THE NATURAL HIGH

Emotional addiction doesn't just apply to negative feelings—it can also work in a positive manner and benefit our health. One way to influence this is through regular movement. Exercise causes our bodies to release feel-good chemicals and hormones, but since that high eventually goes away, we'll keep going back for more—we'll continue to seek the next big thrill.

Regular exercise does wonders to elevate our mood and can help establish more positive or happy emotions as our default. It also helps us to wake up feeling generally upbeat on a regular basis and increases the chance that we carry that mood with us throughout the day. You won't make a big deal out of small things, and your thoughts, actions, and behaviors will be congruent with that feeling of happiness.

Ideally, we want our default setting to be one with healthy

behaviors, thoughts, and attitudes. We're human, and we will fluctuate here and there, but we always want to return to a solid baseline of health—it's important to keep moving, eating well, and working on the mind.

INACTIVITY AND MOOD

A negative emotional setting can have a detrimental effect and drastically impact your health. To give an example, my father was very active until a spinal cord cyst meant he had to stop working. He went from moving around all the time to becoming completely inactive due to the pain, and over time, it distinctly changed his mood and cognition. His situation changed his emotions, and he often felt down and depleted— his previous, healthier attitudes and behaviors no longer influenced his thoughts.[44]

INFLUENCING BRAINWAVES

To keep our overall health in optimal balance, we can't just take care of the body—we also need to take care of the brain. They are both integral parts of the same entity, and the health of one directly influences the health of the other. *Brain waves* are synchronized electrical pulses that facilitate communication between groups of neurons.

---

44 Fernando Lopes da Silva, "Neural Mechanisms Underlying Brain Waves: From Neural Membranes to Networks," *Electroencephalography and Clinical Neurophysiology*, 79, no. 2 (August 1991): 81-93. https://doi.org/10.1016/0013-4694(91)90044-5.

They're associated with conscious brain activity, and we actually have the power to influence their effectiveness. In this section, we'll discuss four types of brain waves: beta, alpha, theta, and delta.

BETA WAVES

Beta brain waves are a dominant part of our lives. They range in frequency from low to high, with lower levels being ideal. When at a lower frequency, these brain waves facilitate logic, reason, planning, learning, and concentration.[45] Because of this, functioning in beta wave frequency is ideal for most waking hours of the day. We want to be in "low beta" each day with a clear focus. However, stress can cause these waves to move at a higher frequency, causing us to function in a less-than-ideal state.

Let's say you start the day feeling relaxed and calm, but then you're late to pick up the kids, you miss a dentist appointment, and you get a bill that you weren't expecting; then, you eat crap food and run out of time to exercise. All of this stress builds up, and the frequency of your beta waves increases through the course of the day.

As the frequency increases, logic and reason decrease, and

---

45   Ranganatha Sitaram et al., "Closed-Loop Brain Training: The Science of Neurofeedback," *National Review of Neuroscience* 18, no. 2 (February 2017): 86–100. https://doi.org/10.1038/nrn.2016.164.

feelings of tension and anxiety rise—you may have exaggerated reactions or inappropriate responses to certain matters.[46] For example, you might lose your temper over your kid doing something as simple as spilling a glass of milk, and nobody wants to feel this way. To make matters worse, remaining in a state of "high beta" for prolonged periods of time means that you're experiencing low-grade chronic stress, which we know leads to chronic illness. For many of us, we start our day in the higher beta frequency, often a continuation from the day before due to a lack of deep sleep.

Consider how this may affect your ability to make changes in your life. When we experience a higher state of stress, even just a little, it rarely results in more logical and sensible decision making. It's crucial for your performance throughout the day to start and maintain an ideal brain wave frequency.

ALPHA WAVES

Next, we have alpha waves. These are of a lower frequency than beta waves, and we often experience them during periods of daydreaming and relaxation—it's an "economy frequency" of a brainwave.[47] That said, it's good for us to be in an alpha state to help decrease stress and

46   Ibid.

47   Ibid.

boost immunity. You can generally keep alpha waves in check, but periodic deep breathing exercises along with meditation are tremendously helpful in producing and maintaining these waves.[48]

THETA WAVES

Theta waves are even slower than alpha waves, and they allow us to connect with our subconscious.[49] These waves are associated with a spiritual space where we can influence the subconscious mind to create our reality. Theta waves are beneficial to our health, and they are essential to creating a new version of ourselves.

DELTA WAVES

Delta brainwaves are the slowest, lowest frequency waves, produced during deep meditation and sleep—they relax and calm us.[50] Deep sleep is vitally important due to the production of these waves, and also because it's when most of our body's growth and repair occurs: immune func-

48 Kok Suen Cheng, Ray P.S. Han, and Poh Foong Lee, "Neurophysiological Study on the Effect of Various Short Duration of Deep Breathing: A Randomized Controlled Trial," *Respiratory Physiology and Neurobiology* 249 (February 2018): 23–31. https://doi.org/10.1016/j.resp.2017.12.008.

49 Bruce Stinson and David Arthur, "A Novel EEG for Alpha Brain State Training, Neurobiofeedback, and Behavior Change," *Complementary Therapies in Clinical Practice* 19, no. 3 (August 2013): 114–8. https://doi.org/10.1016/j.ctcp.2013.03.003.

50 Robert T. Thibault, Michael Lifshitz, and Amir Raz, "The Self-Regulating Brain and Neurofeedback: Experimental Science and Clinical Promise," *Cortex* 74 (January 2016): 247–61. https://doi.org/10.1016/j.cortex.2015.10.024.

tions go to work, and human growth hormone is released.[51] Delta waves also refresh and prepare us for the next day—they help us to feel energized when we wake up.

Delta waves are imperative to rest and repair, which is why FIT 5-40-5 encourages deep meditation at the end of the day—it brings us into a state of relaxation and gratitude, and it creates an easier transition into this wave frequency.

MINDFULNESS WITH FIT 5-40-5

The FIT 5-40-5 mindfulness component emphasizes mental strength and acuity. To begin rewiring your brain and producing the mental state most conducive to change, we suggest completing a brief meditation and breathing exercise each day. This should be done at least once per day, but can be used at any point if you feel stress levels rising, or simply as a mid-day relaxation technique. Our sequence is a short 5-minute meditation, followed by 40 seconds of deep breathing, and completed with another 5-minute meditation.

Morning meditations focus more on preparing you for the day. They involve creating your ideal day through visualization, and feeling and experiencing the emotions

---

51 Richard J. Davidson et al., "Alterations in Brain and Immune Function Produced by Mindfulness Meditation," *Psychosomatic Medicine* 65, no. 4 (July-August 2003): 564–70. https://doi.org/10.1097/01.psy.0000077505.67574.e3.

associated with that day. Evening meditations focus on relaxation, healing, and gratitude—you'll reconnect with yourself and tie into your subconscious. These are ideal for bringing you into a balanced state, making it easier for you to fall into a deep sleep.

Anyone working to create change should spend more time meditating and connecting with their subconscious, at least at the beginning of the process, because that's where the imprint of change happens. At the very least you should be using these techniques to unwind and relax. However, using these techniques should be in alignment with your desired change.

There is no one-size-fits-all approach to fitness and movement, and the same applies to mindfulness. This is why the FIT 5-40-5 program offers a lot of versatility. One of the most common objections we hear from people about meditation is that they don't have time for it. We developed our system to address this objection by making meditations as short and efficient as possible without losing any of the great benefits associated with the practice.

If you can't spare ten minutes in a day, we urge you to reflect and ask yourself, "If somebody watched me for an entire day, would they find ten minutes of spare time?" If we're being honest with ourselves, the answer is most likely, yes, they would. Maybe a modest change in routine is required to make the time, such as going to bed ten minutes later, waking up ten minutes earlier, or possibly spending ten minutes of quiet over your lunch time. If you find you are unwilling to do the work, then it most likely means you're not fully committed to change. However, it's not difficult to get started. The FIT 5-40-5 mindfulness protocol is flexible; you choose what works for you with respect to the timing of the guided meditations, visualizations, and breathing exercises.

For example, it's important for me to do a mid-day visualization and breathing technique to make sure I'm not increasing my beta frequency—I want to maintain logic and reason throughout the day, which is crucial because of my busy schedule. By doing this, it helps me keep my emotions in balance as I work through my usually eventful days.

Ryan, on the other hand, prefers doing a single meditation sequence in the evening shortly before bed. He likes to reflect on the day and prepare himself for a deep sleep. Growth and repair is particularly important to him because his favorite pastime is hiking the Scottish Highlands, often for hours on end. As a personal preference, he does our FIT 5-40-5 mindfulness sequence at the summit of each Munro he climbs, where he finds it therapeutic to connect with nature to balance out his regularly hectic workdays.

Typically, we experience the highest levels of stress during the workweek. These days are filled with repetitive behaviors, and it's common for us to have little or no variety in our days—it's the same routine, day in and day out. In fact, the majority of the thoughts we have on any given day are the same thoughts we had the day before. In fact, the National Science Foundation published an article highlighting this. The article stated that the average person will have twelve thousand to sixty thousand thoughts per day. It went on to suggest that 80 percent of these thoughts are negative and approximately 95 percent of our thoughts would be the same as the day before.[52]

Even if we are physically unable to have a variety of new experiences, we can still create change through our thoughts—we can have the emotions associated with an experience, and the brain won't know the difference between thoughts and reality. We're creating the wiring and chemical connection in our brain for the act before we even carry it out.

THE POWER OF THE MIND

When some people hear the term "meditation," they may

---

52 Hui-Xia Zhou et al., "Rumination and the Default Mode Network: Meta-Analysis of Brain Imaging Studies and Implications for Depression," *NeuroImage* 206 (February 2020). https://doi.org/10.1016/j.neuroimage.2019.116287.

feel intimidated, especially if they don't know much about it. Younger generations are certainly more familiar with it, and it is second nature in many Eastern philosophies, but the Western world has yet to fully embrace this practice. Even if you aren't aiming for the highest level of spiritual being, there is still great value in meditation.

On any given day, meditation can produce beneficial physiological payoffs, including creating an efficient stress response, decreasing cortisol production, and increasing the release of HGH. And this might possibly be the best benefit of all: meditation can increase the length of our telomeres and lower our biological age. One study showed that "short-term meditators" had a biological age that was five years lower than those who were considered "non-meditators." Those are exceptional results!

FOREVER YOUNG

Our physiological age is not always the same as our chronological age. This explains why some people thrive at the age of sixty, while others struggle. We can't do anything about getting older, but we have significant control over our biological age. Movement, proper nutrition, and practicing mindfulness can help us stay biologically young.

What happens in your mind influences every cell of your body. For example, controlling your thoughts and emotions can help keep your hormones in check. Hormones always work within the circumstances of the body, and when they are produced in optimal amounts, you create optimal health.

TRANSFORMATION THROUGH FIT 5-40-5

We begin our program with a ninety-day progression to allow plenty of time for behaviors and attitudes to transform. After ninety days, you'll continue your life as the "new version" of you, with appropriate health goals and challenges in place. (See Appendix G for an audio link to sample meditations.)

CHAPTER 6

////////////

OVERCOMING ROADBLOCKS AND CHALLENGES

The hardest times often lead to the greatest moments of your life. Keep going. Tough situations build strong people in the end.

—ROY T. BENNETT

Despite the routine nature of our lives, they can be exciting, rewarding, demanding, challenging, and full of opportunity. With all that life holds, it can be overwhelming to begin taking steps toward change. In this chapter, we will discuss some common roadblocks to goal achievement, offer tips and advice to help you move closer to health and wellness, and to make the most of the time that you have.

ROADBLOCK #1: WE'RE TOO BUSY

According to James McCourt, owner of Hidden Depths Coaching, the most common reason why people fail is that they never *start*. That simple tenet applies to everyone, from a young child learning to ride a bike, to a legendary athlete at the top of their game. Wayne Gretzky, arguably the greatest hockey player of all time, summed it up well when he said, "You miss 100 percent of the shots you don't take."

Since life is busy and it moves quickly, we often think we don't have time to learn or do something new. However, if you want to accomplish something, you have to make a commitment to yourself that you will work toward it. The process may be slow, and you'll most likely encounter challenges along the way, but you have to give yourself the opportunity to begin.

To start, you need to dissect your day, assign value to everything you do, and make the time to prioritize your health. It's really not that difficult to find squandered time, and once you find it, you can fill it with productive activity.

ROADBLOCK #2: WE DON'T PLAN

As the old adage says, "Fail to Plan, Plan to Fail." Most people who have tried to make significant change in themselves and their circumstances are well aware it doesn't happen by chance. Those people who can consistently get the results they set out to achieve have strategies and plans in place. They know how to set goals, determine milestones along the way to gauge whether or not they are on the right path, and proceed with their plans. Before you start taking the physical action steps to create a change, be sure to remember that you can't skip the planning phase. This will provide clarity of what you want to achieve and what you need to do in order to achieve it. One of the more effective ways to make your plan is to reverse engineer the process by starting with the end in mind. The practice allows you to work backwards from your endpoint and identify all the things you will need to have accomplished prior to that goal becoming a reality. Using this strategy, you can implement time frames for achieving specific milestones that will need to be achieved along the path to achieving your ultimate outcome. Make your plan then work your plan!

ROADBLOCK #3: WE MAKE EXCUSES

Excuses are disempowering, and often hold us back from achieving our goals. They also give us a reason to avoid responsibility for our choices or actions. However, the more knowledge we have, the fewer excuses we will make. When we know we can be held accountable or responsible for an outcome, and we know the reason *why* an outcome is desirable, we're less likely to try and avoid it. We recommend an accountability partner to help if you are inclined to make excuses. Some people are very good at convincing themselves that their excuse is actually a legitimate reason for not sticking to their plan. This is where an accountability partner comes in. Someone you can check in with regularly that knows your plan, is aware of your goal, and understands your reason for doing it—your WHY! Have an accountability partner who you know won't let you off easy. This shouldn't be that friend who can convince you to go for a cocktail instead of a workout.

ROADBLOCK #4: WE'RE UNAWARE

Lack of awareness is another factor that holds us back. Some people don't know what they can do to change, and some unhealthy people may think they don't need to change at all. For instance, not everybody knows what a healthy diet looks like, and some might think that they are eating healthy, when in fact, they aren't.

Other people may question whether or not they can commit to the activities that are required to change their lifestyle. It's easy to overestimate what we think it takes to become healthy, particularly when it comes to exercise. We constantly see advertisements for fast abs and twenty-minute training, and social media posts from fitness gurus and boot camps seem to be in our faces all the time. The level of training depicted in those ads is fantastic for people who are chasing a high level of fitness, but the physical demand isn't that high for someone who simply wants to be healthy.

A HEALTHY PERSPECTIVE

When we put our health at the forefront of our lives, much of our stress goes away, the body's chemistry improves, and we can work our way back to homeostasis. Unfortunately, many of us experience chronic stress, and we don't focus on our health until we are facing illness or disease. Instead of treating the pathology (the disease or diagnosis), we need to correct the problems that got us there in the first place. The FIT 5-40-5 program addresses these issues and helps to restore homeostasis in the body.

If we look at life from a disease perspective, we never really win because we're only treating the disease and its symptoms. But if we start looking at health as the by-product of every choice we make and everything we put into our bodies, we can develop habits to establish and maintain it. Almost every chronic disease we face today is the result of physiological changes in the body due to chemical, physical, or emotional stress. If we want to thrive, we can't just focus on treating diabetes, heart disease, or cancer; we have to focus on promoting health by emphasizing the lifestyle factors that will help us return to homeostasis.

PERSIST TO CHANGE

It takes about thirty days of repetition of an activity to "hardwire" or change the neurological pattern in the brain. When we say "hardwire," we mean the imprinting of new beliefs, actions, or behaviors, while simultaneously letting go of old ones. If you are genuinely committed to making a lasting change, seeing a difference in yourself, and creating a new reality, then be consistent over time. Taking a break in your transformation opens the door to reintroducing the old, unwanted beliefs and behaviors. More often than not, the door doesn't get shut again. You need to be consistent, and you need to give it time. It is true that change can happen in a moment, but results do take time. This is why it's so important to continue a behavior consistently for at least a month: you want to give your brain a chance to adjust to a new neurological pattern. As this new pattern develops, things become easier. The voice of the "devil on the shoulder" trying to convince you to skip your meditation, go for a cocktail instead of the gym, or to put the tub of ice cream in your shopping basket becomes weaker and weaker until it can no longer be heard—it's not you anymore.

ARE YOU TRULY HEALTHY?

If we were to ask a group of people at random what they thought about their health, many would say, "Oh, I'm good," "Pretty healthy," "It's reasonable," or "I'm healthy."

Some might be answering truthfully, and others might be unaware of the reality of their health status. We attribute this to a combination of overconfidence, denial, and ignorance. When someone drops dead from a heart attack, the common reaction is shock and surprise, naturally. However, we are surprised by how often we hear people describing the deceased as having been "fit as a fiddle" or being "fit and healthy!" Of course, that wasn't really the case. Heart disease manifests slowly over time, and it doesn't necessarily carry symptoms. In fact, many first-time heart attacks result in death, and at that point it's too late to heed the warning of heart disease.

How many people today are diagnosed with cancer? How many of those people do you think went in for a routine check-up expecting a normal report, and they were told, "We found something alarming—we need to run some tests." All of those people thought they were healthy, when in fact they had a disease developing in their body. Don't wait until it takes you forever to walk down the driveway, your knees hurt from climbing the stairs, or you get a little winded while walking to the store. Please don't gamble with your health. The time to take action is *now*.

Take a moment to assess your behaviors over the last month. Are you exercising regularly? Are you drinking alcohol every Friday night, or worse, every night? Are you eating fast food once a week, or even once a day? Based on your current lifestyle, will your health be better or worse five, ten, or twenty years from now? Consider which behaviors you should continue, and which ones you need to change. If you aren't creating the right circumstances for a long and healthy life, you need to do something about it today. See Appendix E for our Reality Health Checklist.

CONCLUSION

You can't afford to get sick, and you can't depend on the present healthcare system to keep you well. It's up to you to protect and maintain your body's innate capacity for health and healing by making the right choices in how you live.

—ANDREW WEIL

If you only take away one thing from this book, it should be the fact that you were born with an intelligent body. You were not designed by chance: that intelligence created you, works within you every day, and it will never stop. When you get sick or battle injury, that intelligence constantly works to heal you. In all manifestations and expressions of health or stress, the body adapts its physiology to keep you alive as best it can.

We don't know of any of our colleagues who would disagree with what we stated above. Healthcare providers of all types can play an important role in our lives and intervene at various levels of sickness. However, we guarantee that almost all of them would agree that many of their patients (you) would not be sick in the first place if they had taken better care of themselves.

EMPOWERED TO CHANGE

With sedentary jobs and external stressors being more prevalent today, movement, proper nutrition, and mindfulness are much more essential to your health. Life is expensive, people don't like their jobs, and the world is a tumultuous place to raise kids; the challenges are real, but you must make a shift if you want to enjoy life for as long as possible.

If you're not doing the things that you could or should be doing to move toward health and wellness, that's unfortunate. However, there's a light at the end of the tunnel: you can take control of your health at any stage in life. We believe that everyone wants to change and get better, but some don't know where to begin, or they don't know what is required to facilitate that change. For a full innate transformation, you must break old patterns, form new habits through repetition, and establish the "why" behind your everyday choices. In order to become a new person, you need to begin thinking and living like the person you want to be and FIT 5-40-5 can help you do just that.

The goal of the program is to empower you and help minimize the roadblocks on your journey, and we do this through our adaptable and flexible program design. If you find that our program isn't what you are looking for, there are other programs out there that are equally fantastic. Find one that resonates with you, so you can begin moving closer to your end goal of better health and wellness.

MAKE THE CHOICE

Please don't be intimidated at the thought of making a change. Countless people have made life-changing transformations, and it's well within your grasp to do the same. The body is amazing and powerful, even if your goal may seem a long way off in the moment, your body is up to the challenge. With a little bit of encouragement and assistance, you can turn things around. If you make every effort to minimize stress and maintain balance and homeostasis, the results will manifest in your body.

Remember, excuses and blame disempower while action and planning serve to empower. When you set a goal, you need to have a clear destination, and don't allow roadblocks to get in your way. Having a clear vision makes it easier to navigate the journey.

Exercise, nutrition, and mindfulness are key to achieving optimal health, but you must also remind yourself on a daily basis that you are grateful to be alive. Take the time to relax and enjoy being you. Reflect upon what's happening in your life and bring yourself back into balance. Let yourself get excited about wellness and make the decision to change your life.

APPENDICES

The mantra in our clinics and our business is to move, feel, and live better. When you move more, feeling and living better happen naturally as a result. Everything in our program is achievable, from the beginner to advanced level. Find a FIT 5-40-5 healthcare partner near you and join our community. More information is available at www. fit5-40-5.com.

The following appendices can help you along your wellness journey. Be sure to try the sample 3-DAY FIT 5-40-5 Challenge at the end of this section.

////////////

SELF-TEST FOR PROPRIOCEPTION

The following are instructions to follow which will allow you to test your own proprioception, your sixth sense. Proprioception has a crucial role to play in balance, coordination, movement, muscle tone, and posture. It's easy to see why it is important to have an optimum proprioceptive feedback loop from the body to brain and back to our body. Equally important, as discussed in the book, is the relationship between proprioception and our moods/emotions. Here are a couple quick tests to check your proprioception. You will see from your results if this is something that you might need to focus on.

TEST #1

First, try the one we mentioned in the book. Close your eyes, close your fists, only leaving one finger on each hand extended.

Reach your arms behind your back and try to touch the two extended fingertips together.

How accurate were you on your first try? You should be able to hit the fingertips together without any problem at all.

TEST #2

Now, this next test is a little bit more involved. It's best to do it with someone in case you need support with balance.

Find an open space. You want to use some white, black, or colored tape and tape the capital letter T on the floor. The T should be about a meter long and a meter wide across the top.

Your starting position is standing at the top of the T with your heels on the line on each side facing down the line to the bottom of the T.

Hold your arms out in front of you at 90 degrees to your shoulder with your palms facing up to the ceiling. Look straight ahead. Begin marching on the spot with high knees for 20 seconds.

Have your partner time you. They can tell you when 20 seconds is up. Stop with both feet on the ground. Once you have stopped marching, have a look down and take note of any movement forward or backward or deviation side to side away from your start position. That's part 1 of this test. Make a note if you had any movement.

Go back to your start position. You will repeat the same test, only this time you must close your eyes. This is when it is very important you have someone standing by your side for support if needed.

Begin marching with high knees on the spot, and don't open your eyes. Remember to keep your arms out in front with your palms up to the ceiling. Continue marching on the spot for 20 seconds. This time, when your partner tells you to stop, don't open your eyes yet. Tell your partner how much you think you have moved, if at all. Then open your eyes.

If there was more movement this time without the use of your eyes, then you may have poor proprioception. How much depends on how much you moved. With an optimum proprioceptive feedback loop, you should be pretty much as good with your eyes open as you are when they are closed.

*Remember, when doing this test, you must get your knees up when you march, and it should be the same style of marching with your eyes open and closed.

How is your proprioception?

APPENDIX B

//////////////

THE CORE 40 FOOD GUIDE

FIT 5-40-5 CORE 40 FOODS

AISLE 1 *LEAFY GREEN VEG*	AISLE 2 *VEGETABLES*	AISLE 3 *ANIMAL*	AISLE 4 *NUTS & SEEDS*	AISLE 5 *FRUITS & BERRIES*
Spinach	Asparagus	Eggs	Almond	Tomato
Kale	Cucumber	Chicken	Brazil	Banana
Rocket Arugula	Carrot	Lamb	Walnut	Orange
Broccoli	Zucchini	Beef	Hazelnut	Avocado
Watercress	Onion	Game	Pecan	Apple
Cauliflower	Bell Pepper	Salmon	Sunflower Seed	Blueberry
Romaine Lettuce	Mushroom	Sea Bass	Pumpkin Seed	Strawberry
Swiss Chard	Celery	Pork	Chia Seed	Raspberry

THE PANTRY *(OILS, CONDIMENTS, ETC.)*

Fats & Oils: Extra Virgin Olive Oil, Coconut Oil, Avocado Oil, Hemp Oil, Sesame Oil, Organic Butter, Nut Oils (cold-pressed, not for cooking)

Spreads/Butters/Sauces: Almond Butter, Hummus, Raw Honey, Tahini, Jars of Olives, Apple Cider Vinegar, Dijon Mustard, Mayonnaise, Coconut Milk, Balsamic, Soy Sauce (Tamari = Gluten Free)

Herbs and Spices: Garlic, Ginger, Tumeric, Cumin, Cinnamon, Black Pepper, Lemon, Lime, Sea Salt (or Himalayan), Bouillon Vegetable Stock

Beverages: Organic Ground Coffee, Green Tea, Peppermint Tea, Any Herbal Teas

Cheese/Dairy: Halloumi, Goat Cheese, Feta, Greek Yogurt (Natural)

Milk Alternative: Oat Milk (best in tea and coffee), Almond, Hemp

Extras: Dark Chocolate (85%), Olives

Fermented Foods: Fermented Veggies, Kimchi, Sauerkraut, Apple-Cider Vinegar

////////////

LIST OF RECOMMENDED SUPPLEMENTS

Multivitamins and mineral supplements.

Omega 3 Oil—Best sources are DHA/EPA, from wild fish or Algae (vegan option).

Magnesium—Approximately 500mg per day. **Note:** If you have any kidney disease or issues with your kidneys, you must consult your physician first to find out if supplementing with magnesium is safe for you.

Vitamin D3—Oil or tablet form are both acceptable. Take 400-500 international units (IUs) per day. More is acceptable during the winter if you live in the northern hemisphere. If you don't get 15-20 minutes of sunlight per day on over 50 percent of your body (bare skin), then you should consider supplementing with vitamin D3.

Vitamin K2-4/K2-9

Greens Powder—Look for a comprehensive formula with a diverse range of green vegetable powders. Go for organic where possible.

Meal Replacement Powder—Plant-based protein powder combined with other nourishing ingredients, including vitamins and minerals to provide a complete option for a meal replacement (e.g., FullyIn8 Meal Replacement).

APPENDIX D

//////////////

GOAL SETTING

When setting goals, it is important to be as detailed as possible. For example, saying "I want to lose weight" isn't clear enough. Losing just one pound would satisfy that statement. Therefore, setting a goal about weight loss should specify the amount of weight you want to lose and by what date. The more specific you can be, then the easier it is to make your plan and work your plan.

So, before we begin the process of setting a goal, take the time to think about your life. What do you want to experience and accomplish? What old habits do you want to replace with new ones that will help you live better and more fulfilled? What areas of your life do you want to improve? Write this down. Once you have finished, take the time to reflect on what you have put down and make sure these statements are about you. Are they realistic?

Are they achievable? For example, saying you want to lose 200 pounds in one month is not achievable. Use the following steps:

1. Make your goal statement.
2. How will this goal benefit your life?
3. What is your timeline for achieving your goal?

Next, set your action plan:

1. What actions do you need to take in order to achieve this goal (be specific)?
2. What are you doing already that will help you achieve this goal?
3. What actions and behaviors must you change in order to achieve your goal?
4. Set milestones to assess your progress. What needs to be achieved by when in order to ensure you are on track to achieve your goals in the desired time frame?
5. Ask yourself if anything to this point in your plan seems unrealistic. If it is, revise it. If it is not, then proceed.
6. Schedule your action plan. Be as detailed as possible. At what times will you eat? What time of day will you exercise? What time of day will you meditate? Be as detailed as you can, scheduling and accounting for each action step in your plan.
7. Finally, choose an accountability partner. Choose

someone who understands the importance of you achieving your goal and is strong enough not to accept your excuses along the way. The accountability partner can be a make or break for some people, especially if you are in the habit of making excuses. Choose wisely.

8. Stick to your plan.

//////////

REALITY HEALTH CHECKLIST

Answer the following questions with either **YES** or **NO**:

CARDIOVASCULAR

Do I...

...get chest pain when performing normal activities? _____

...have a feeling of irregular or "skipped" heartbeat? _____

...get a rapid or pounding heartbeat? _____

...find that my legs get puffy or swollen frequently? _____

...feel dizzy when getting up from a sitting or lying position? _____

RESPIRATORY

Do I...

...feel short of breath when walking upstairs or going for a walk? _____

...often have cold hands/feet? _____

...often suffer from a cough? _____

...sound wheezy when taking normal or deep breaths? _____

DIGESTIVE

Do I...

...often feel bloated? _____

...have the appearance of a swollen abdomen? _____

...pass gas frequently? _____

...have unpleasant-smelling breath? _____

...often have pain in the stomach or intestinal area? _____

ENDOCRINE

Do I...

...regularly suffer from fatigue/lethargy? _____

...excessively sweat, even when not exerting myself? _____

...have crashes in my energy after eating? _____

...struggle to lose weight even through calorie restriction? _____

...suffer from acne, dry, or itchy skin? _____

IMMUNE

Do I...

...take antibiotics for infections frequently (more than once per year)? _____

...suffer from hay fever or other allergies?

...regularly have a runny nose or frequent sneezing?

...always seem to catch a cold or flu? _____

...have excessive mucus in the throat or nose? _____

NERVOUS SYSTEM

Do I...

...often lose my balance or struggle with coordination (feel clumsy)? _____

...have poor memory or often feel confused? _____

...struggle to concentrate on even simple tasks? _____

...get angry or irritable quite easily? _____

...feel restless when trying to sleep? _____

...have fluctuating moods? _____

MUSCULOSKELETAL

Do I...

...get sore in my knees, ankles and/or back while walking up a flight of stairs?

...get regular joint pain and/or stiffness? _____

...have limited range of movement (i.e., difficulty bending to tie my shoes or looking over my shoulder while driving)? _____

...feel tired after a small amount of exercise? _____

...feel weak while doing a minor amount of exercise? _____

...struggle to lift objects (the kettle, pots/pans, etc.?) _____

Total # of YES Answers _____

Total # of NO Answers _____

APPENDIX F

////////////

LIST OF HELPFUL WEBSITES

www.fit5-40-5.com

www.familyhealthadvocacy.com

www.FullyIn8.com

www.draxe.com

www.standardprocess.com

www.drjoedispenza.com

www.jamesmccourt.co.uk

////////////

THE FIT 5-40-5, 3-DAY CHALLENGE

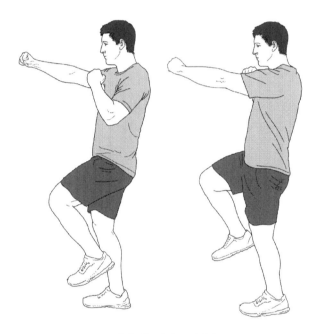

1.1. Sprint and Jabs

1.2. Air Squat

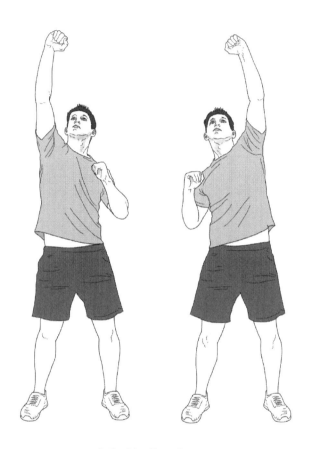

1.3. Sky Punches

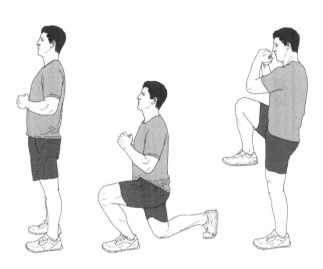

1.4. Step Back High Knee

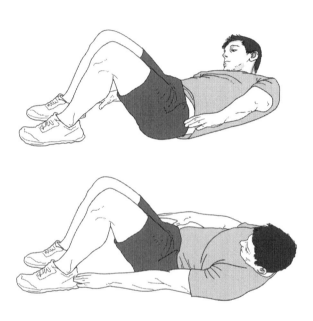

1.5. Heel Touches

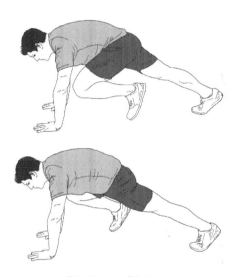

2.1. Mountain Climbers

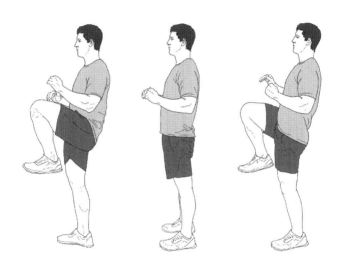

2.2. High Knees

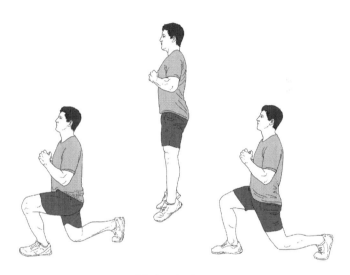

2.3. Jumping Lunges

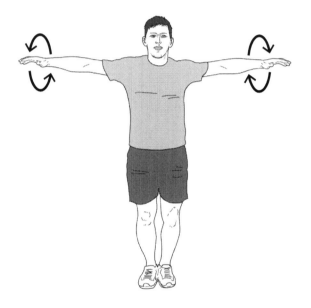

2.4. Fast Arm Circles

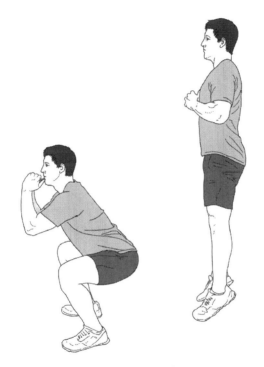

2.5. Jumping Squat

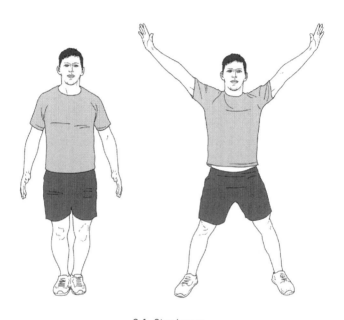

3.1. Star Jumps

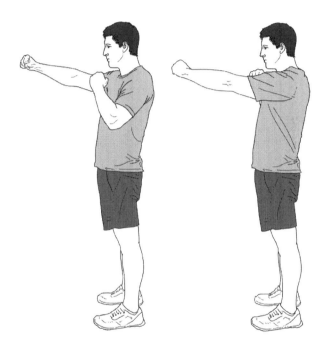

3.2. Standing Jabs

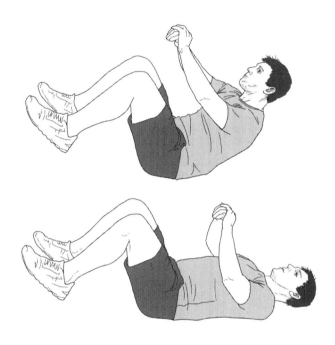

3.3. Crunch

3.4. Press Up

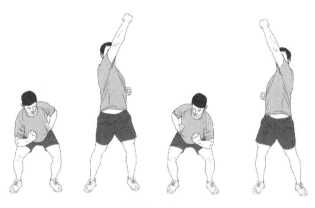

3.5. Upper Cuts

3-DAY MEAL PLAN

DAY 1	DAY 2	DAY 3
Breakfast Bacon & Avocado Bowl	*Breakfast* Yogurt & Blueberries	*Breakfast* Nut & Berry Smoothie
Lunch Spinach, Feta & Walnut Salad	*Lunch* Tomato & Pesto Salad	*Lunch* Chicken Salad
Dinner Wilted Greens & Salmon	*Dinner* Chicken & Asparagus	*Dinner* Beef Stir Fry

SNACK OPTIONS

These can be eaten between Breakfast and Lunch, or Lunch and Dinner.
These are:

- 25g Dark Chocolate, 85%
- Selection of Raw Veg (cucumber, carrot, asparagus, pepper, celery) dipped in Hummus. Shop-bought (organic where possible) or homemade is suitable
- 80g Mixed Olives
- 1–2 Pieces of Fruit from Core 40
- Mixed Berries, 50–80g

Use the following link to get access to the audio files for the meditations for this 3-Day Challenge. When doing your meditation, be sure to find a quiet, calm place where you can relax without distractions or interruptions for ten to fifteen minutes.

https://fit5-40-5.com/free-meditations

ENJOY!

ACKNOWLEDGMENTS

To all of the participants and patients who took part in the early days of FIT 5-40-5, we would like to thank you for trusting us with assisting in your health transformations. Your willingness to be open, committed, and dedicated to the process has inspired us to continue to grow the program and help more people realize their health potential.

James McCourt, we would like to thank you for sharing your thoughts and wisdom with respect to the mindfulness component to this program and book. Your guidance was instrumental in helping us understand the repeated behavioral patterns we were seeing along the way in our patients. This was invaluable in the refinement of our program and will help us as we progress and develop FIT 5-40-5 to greater levels.

Dr. Ed Osburn, thank you for introducing us to the power of virtual business. You helped guide our vision of moving our program from our small premises to the online world. This process has allowed us to expand our potential to help more people beyond what we thought was possible.

Dr. Jason Richardson, we are grateful for your instant support, interest, and participation in the development process of the FIT 5-40-5 program. We are flattered and inspired by your positive critique of FIT 5-40-5. On a personal note, your mindset coaching helped us break barriers we had set between the ears.

To Kiran Dunne and David McCourt, thank you for allowing us to share your stories in our book. Your stories will help people see what's possible. To see the transformations you have both made is remarkable. We are honored to work with you both.

ABOUT THE AUTHORS

GAVIN SINCLAIR was raised to embrace a natural approach to health and well-being. As a second-generation chiropractor, Gavin studied community health science at Brock University in Canada and later obtained his Master of Chiropractic degree in England. Gavin currently operates four private-practice clinics in Scotland, and since 2006, he has been educating patients on the roles that proper exercise, nutrition, and a healthy mind play in promoting optimal health.

RYAN COPLESTON'S interest in health and wellness began early in childhood when he made a very personal transformation in his own life. Learning what was needed to change his health led him down a path that resulted in him graduating as a chiropractor in 2017 and moving to Scotland to practice. His passion lies in helping individuals transform their health so that they can get the most enjoyment from life.